PERSONALITY AND PSYCHOTHERAPY

Personality and Psychotherapy
Treating the Whole Person

JEFFERSON A. SINGER

THE GUILFORD PRESS
New York   London

For Anne, Olivia, and Chloe

© 2005 The Guilford Press
A Division of Guilford Publications, Inc.
72 Spring Street, New York, NY 10012
www.guilford.com

Printed in the United States of America

This book is printed on acid-free paper.

Last digit is print number: 9 8 7 6 5 4 3 2 1

Library of Congress Cataloging-in-Publication Data

Singer, Jefferson A.
   Personality and psychotherapy : treating the whole person / Jefferson A. Singer.
      p. cm.
   Includes bibliographical references and index.
   ISBN 1-59385-211-8
   1. Client-centered psychotherapy. I. Title.
   RC481.S54 2005
   616.89′14—dc22

                                                            2005010751

About the Author

Jefferson A. Singer, PhD, is a professor of psychology at Connecticut College in New London, Connecticut, and a clinical psychologist with a private practice in Waterford, Connecticut. He has written two previous books, *The Remembered Self: Emotion and Memory in Personality* (with Peter Salovey) and *Message in a Bottle: Stories of Men and Addiction*, as well as numerous articles, chapters, and reviews on clinical psychology and personality and memory. Dr. Singer is a fellow of the American Psychological Association, past associate editor of the *Journal of Personality*, and the 2005 recipient of the Theodore R. Sarbin Award for Theoretical Contributions to Psychology, presented by Division 24 (Theoretical and Philosophical Psychology) of the American Psychological Association. Dr. Singer lives in West Hartford, Connecticut, with his wife, Anne, and their two daughters, Olivia and Chloe.

Preface

I hope in this book to fill a major gap in the training and knowledge base of psychotherapists, including clinical psychologists, counseling psychologists, psychiatrists, social workers, and marriage and family counselors. Training in these fields has not kept up with rapid advances in the field of personality psychology in the last 20 years. Just as we have seen remarkable progress in neuroscience and cognitive science, there have been significant strides made in the study of personality that have left older textbooks obsolete and many current ones no longer cutting-edge. Yet even the most up-to-date textbooks in personality are not designed to connect the research they describe to the needs and concerns of the practicing therapist.

The goal of this volume is to help therapists, therapists-in-training, and the instructors in charge of their training close this gap and become familiar with some of the most important contemporary personality research. By providing case material drawn from research participants as well as clients from my own practice, I demonstrate the relevance and utility of personality psychology for the understanding and effective treatment of clients in psychotherapy. To accomplish this endeavor, I take readers systematically through Dan McAdams's three-domain framework of personality research, which has become a major way of organizing the field of personality psychology. It provides insight into individuals from the perspective of their stable traits (Domain 1); social-cognitive adaptations, such as goals and defenses (Domain 2); and life stories or personal narratives (Domain 3). In addition to these three domains, I also offer readers a review of advances in relational psychotherapy that emphasize the embeddedness of the individual personality in a network of intimate relationships and cultural influences. Throughout the presentation of this material, my main objective is to illustrate its value for a deeper and more insightful understanding of the clients with whom we work in psychotherapy.

This last sentence points to a more philosophical commitment that helps to explain the subtitle of this book—"treating the whole person." In this era of managed care, manualized treatments, and pharmacotherapy, there is still a need for psychotherapy that takes on "problems of living," including the pursuit of self-understanding, improved interpersonal relationships, and the realization of meaning and purpose in one's life. Although these therapeutic challenges do not easily fall into diagnostic categories within the medical model, any working therapist knows that they constitute a large part of the struggles that clients bring to the hours we share with them. Increasingly, therapists feel defensive about this kind of therapeutic activity, which seems somehow less legitimate than the treatment of specified symptoms or biological disorders. To treat an individual's struggle to understand the meaning of a particular memory or to point out ambivalence in the pursuit of a seemingly desirable goal seems less "scientific" or "efficacious" than to provide a set of concrete homework assignments and focused exercises to remediate a symptom. Although there is much value in these latter treatment approaches (and I often employ these strategies in my own work), I am concerned that they are at risk for edging out an equally valid kind of therapy that is more exploratory and meaning-oriented.

Often the grounds for privileging cognitive-behavioral or biological treatments over therapies that focus more on meaning and insight are their adherents' claims of a more solid scientific foundation to support their practice. What I hope to show in this volume is that this conclusion is a misreading of the current scientific evidence. Contemporary personality psychology does in fact provide a strong foundation of research support for therapies that put questions of meaning, self-understanding, and socioemotional growth at the center of their enterprise. Practitioners equipped with the empirical and interpretative advances promulgated by personality psychology need not feel defensive about their commitment to treating the whole person. Although many of us may feel intuitively that such concerns are critical to our purpose as healers, this volume provides an extensive body of research to support this inclination. We should all be grateful for the remarkable achievements that the medical model has brought to the treatment of mental health, but it is also heartening to know that progress continues in the realms of life that lie slightly outside the spheres of disease and disorder. This volume is dedicated to this aspect of therapy—a person-based psychology and psychotherapy that values memories, dreams, life stories, meanings, insights, and relationships in the service of enhanced self-knowledge and quality of life where the end points are often equal measures of happiness and wisdom.

The genesis of this work grew out of conversations with Phyllis Wentworth of Blackwell Press. Although I ended up taking the book in a different direction than we originally envisioned, I am grateful for her suggestion that I write a book that would link my interests in personality psychology and psychotherapy. Seymour Weingarten of The Guilford Press saw the potential that this book might have to meet the needs of practitioners and students to catch up on advances in personality psychology at the same time that they are engaging in a daily fight to defend the person in psychotherapy. Seymour is one of the constant positive influences in the psychology publishing world, and it is simply a statement of fact that my course syllabi continue to be filled with Guilford's titles. Jim Nageotte has been a graceful and gracious editor who has applied thoughtful guidance throughout the process. This book steadily improved under his direction and sensitive scrutiny. Jacquelyn Coggin was an able and exacting copy editor, and Jennifer DePrima provided efficient oversight of the book's production.

In writing a book that takes a position not entirely in sync with the mainstream, it is critical to have colleagues who share your vision of the field and support your efforts to articulate it. I am very much indebted to my fellow members of the Society of Personology, an organization devoted to the study of individuals and their lives. In particular, I am grateful to Nicole Barenbaum, Dan McAdams, and Mac Runyan, who engaged in discussions about and/or reviewed drafts of chapters in this volume that are relevant to their work. I must particularly acknowledge Dan for providing the field with the elegant framework that is the backbone to much of the work presented in the chapters that follow.

A large part of the writing of this book took place over a sabbatical year, generously granted to me by Connecticut College. I am grateful to President Norman Fainstein and Helen Regan and Fran Hoffman, the past and present deans of the faculty, for this privilege. The chair of the psychology department, Stuart Vyse, its administrator, Nancy MacLeod, and the rest of my outstanding departmental colleagues have been a continuing source of support and encouragement throughout the writing process. Other professional colleagues, who are also good friends— Robert Emmons, Robert Giebisch, Gary Greenberg, and Barbara Woike— have been stalwart advisors and supporters. I am blessed to have two friends, Lawrence Vogel of the philosophy department at Connecticut College, and Rand Cooper, a writer, critic, and editor, who live within minutes of my home and who have provided helpful feedback and encouragement throughout every phase of this process.

I am very much indebted to both the United States and United Kingdom Fulbright Commissions for granting me an opportunity to work on writing and research relevant to this book at Durham University in Durham, England. My sponsor was Martin Conway, who was a great source of intellectual stimulation and a wonderful host to my family and me. I am also grateful for the help and friendship of Malcolm Rolling, who oversaw my many different technical and logistical needs during my stay at Durham. Malcolm and the rest of the psychology department staff made sure that I could have a comfortable and quiet space for writing throughout my time there.

This book took shape as I developed and taught a course entitled "Seminar in Personality Research" at Connecticut College in the fall of 2002 and again in the fall of 2004. I owe an incalculable debt to "Jennifer," the student who volunteered to participate in a personality assessment and then agreed to allow her protocol to be used in this volume. I must also acknowledge the meticulous and sensitive work of Natalie McEachern, a student in the fall 2002 seminar, who collected Jennifer's personality data and conducted the initial analyses of her responses. I would like to thank all of the students who took part in these seminars and, in particular the fall 2004 group, who provided invaluable feedback on chapter drafts: Jenna Baddeley, Kate Bogart, Hilary Garrison-Botsford, Liana Guzman, Samantha Lee, Dov Markowitz, Blerim Rexhaj, Alexa Xanthopoulous, and Lydia Willsky. I must especially single out Jenna Baddeley, who has worked as my research assistant on this book. She has been a great sounding board and tireless worker in bringing this project to completion.

Any book that draws on clinical experience owes a huge debt to the clients who provide the actual examples of struggle and insight that make up the psychotherapeutic process. As always, I stand in awe of their strength and courage. An additional acknowledgment must go to "Doug and Karen," the couple who granted me permission to describe their therapy in the final chapter.

Finally, I must thank my family. My parents, Jerome and Dorothy Singer, both psychologists, have served as role models throughout my professional career in their commitment to the integration of research and practice. My brother Bruce, who is currently enrolled in a professional psychology doctoral program and once asked me what might be a good personality book for therapists to read, is certainly a chief inspiration for this book. My oldest brother, Jon, now the only family member who is not a psychologist, has the patience of Job to put up with the monotonous direction that recent family conversations tend to take. Speaking of patience, there must be an infinite supply somewhere that has been tapped by my wife, Anne, and my two daughters, Olivia and Chloe. They have endured countless mornings, evenings, and weekends with the sight of Dad working on yet another draft of "that personality and therapy book" in front of the computer monitor. Each time that I set aside my work to join my life with theirs, I find again the secret to what makes me a whole person and to the fullest meaning and purpose that all of life might offer.

Contents

1

Introduction

The psychology of personality proceeds from the point of view
of the person himself. It asks what *he* is like in his essential
nature. If he is like many things, If he changes from
environment to environment, very well and good. It is always *he*
who changes; and the range and forms of his variations can be
determined. He himself is the datum; he *is* something and *does*
something (or if one prefers, he is *many* things and does *many*
things); but we can still find out what they are viewed from
within, from the person's *own* point of view.
                          —(ALLPORT, 1937, p. 558; emphasis in original)

If you have picked up this book and are reading this first sentence, then it is likely we share a common interest and concern, namely,
that in our sweeping embrace of biological advances and cognitive-
behavioral models, psychology and psychotherapy may be losing sight
of the person. What happens to our efforts to understand an individual's
life as we turn our emphasis more and more to problems of diminished
neural firing or dysfunctional patterns of thoughts? Is there still a *scientific* and *therapeutic* justification for seeing individuals as whole people,
multileveled, complex, and nonreducible to their "working parts"?

This book provides an optimistic and affirmative answer to this
question. Whether you are a therapist or therapist-in-training, the following chapters demonstrate that there is indeed an emerging science of
the person that is relevant to psychotherapy. Even more, this volume illustrates how this person-based science can be directly applied in psychotherapy practice. For personality researchers and graduate students,
this book integrates diverse methods of personality assessment to pro-

1

vide a comprehensive picture of an individual person. For both researchers and therapists, I also review recent advances in relational psychoanalysis that make a strong case for locating individual persons in a
"relational matrix" that takes into account gender, sociocultural influence, and what psychoanalysts would call "shared subjectivities" (if this
last phrase sounds obscure, I promise that I will explain its meaning in
straightforward terms and with concrete examples).

My goal, then, is to build bridges between therapists and scientists
who share a concern for the integrity of the individual person. One
might think that the goal of bringing a person-based psychology to the
attention of clinical psychologists and psychotherapists is a good example of "preaching to the choir." After all, the licensing guidelines for clinical psychology require training programs to offer graduate courses in
personality psychology as one of the core disciplines to be mastered.
However, in my dual career as a professor of psychology and a clinical
psychologist in private practice, I have too often encountered students or
fellow practitioners who think that the field of personality is still encompassed by the original figures of Freud, Jung, and Adler, with a little bit
of Skinner, Rogers, and Maslow thrown in to fill out the picture. Those
with better memories for their course material might mention the social
learning work of Bandura and Mischel, while those inclined toward
measurement remember Cattell's Sixteen Personality Factor Questionnaire (16PF) and factor analysis. Ironically, in light of the increasing
medicalization of psychotherapy, with its emphasis on symptom relief
and disorder, I am actually pleased when a colleague or student expresses some knowledge, however incomplete, about personality psychology. Yet what most therapists out in the field or the vast majority of
students in the typical introductory personality course are not likely to
know is that personality psychology is in the midst of a renaissance. It
has a thriving new international organization, the Association for Research in Personality, that is less than 10 years old, refined instruments
that are being adopted around the world (McCrae, Costa, del Pilar,
Rolland, & Parker, 1998), and theoretical perspectives that have the potential to make integrative connections across the social sciences, health
fields, and humanities (Carver & Scheier, 1998; Conway, Singer, &
Tagini, 2004; Lau, 2002; McAdams, 1999, 2001; Pennebaker, 1995).

As an associate editor for the *Journal of Personality*, one of the major outlets for the publishing of scientific research in personality, I can
attest to our difficulty in keeping up with the volume of submissions of
high-quality research being conducted in personality. This research is
seldom concerned with "psychosexual stages," "archetypes," or "inferiority complexes" (the kinds of terms still encountered in many introduc-

tory personality courses). Instead, contemporary personality researchers ask questions about topics such as the "Big Five," "personal strivings," "social-cognitive strategies," "self-regulation," and "narrative identity," and look at their relationship to "well-being," "optimal adjustment," "agency and communion," and "meaning making." These terms (all of which are covered in this book) are slowly working their way into textbooks on personality, but they are still too new for many therapists or therapists-in-training to have a handle on their meaning or potential application to practice.

The need to address this gap between contemporary personality research and psychotherapy practice became most apparent to me during my tenure in another associate editor position related to clinical psychology. For nearly 5 years, from 1998 to 2003, I served as the associate editor in charge of assigning new clinical psychology books to be reviewed for *Contemporary Psychology: The American Psychological Association's Journal of Book Reviews*. In other words, in the United States, Canada, and the United Kingdom, virtually every book published with any relationship to psychotherapy would arrive on a weekly basis in cartons at my office door, and each year I evaluated 300–400 books for potential review. Of the more than 1,500 books I examined, I would estimate that no more than 10–15 volumes made an explicit link between contemporary personality research and clinical practice. There were many books that drew on contemporary psychoanalytic theory (as well as even more that drew on much older psychoanalytic or psychodynamic theories), but few of these books offered any support other than clinical histories for their assertions. Similarly, there were a smaller number of humanistic and Jungian psychology books that offered complicated discussions of the individual person but were far removed from any link to empirical personality psychology.

A large stock of books, strong in empirical support, applied cognitive-behavioral techniques to specific disorders, ranging from anxiety and depression to eating disorders and addiction. Despite their research base in many aspects of contemporary psychology, these books lacked psychoanalytic and humanistic psychology's sensitivity to a comprehensive vision of the person. To their credit, cognitive-behavioral approaches have traditionally emphasized the reciprocal nature of cognition, behavior, and emotion (Bandura, 1999). Yet the therapies they produce still tend to take a more tinkering or mechanistic perspective that focuses on the malfunctioning components of the person rather than the person as a whole (however, for a more holistic and integrative perspective, see Linehan, 1988; Mahoney, 2003; Segal, Williams, & Teasdale, 2001). In summary, whether looking toward either psychoanalytic and humanistic theory or cognitive-behavioral therapy, it was hard to find a book that was both research-based and concerned with a holistic understanding of the individual person.

Though some of the just-mentioned humanistically oriented psychologists and psychotherapists might still echo Wordsworth's memorable caution, "We murder to dissect" ("The Tables Turned," line 28; Wordsworth, 1798/1984), I propose that we now have the scientific methods to allow us to build a more complete picture of the person without compromising the integrity or multidimensional facets of each individual. Even if you are not inclined to introduce personality inventories or collection of personal memories into your clinical work, this book provides a conceptual framework for how to understand individuals that is likely to be highly relevant to your practice.

However, for those interested in applying the personality instruments described in this book, I give fairly comprehensive introductory descriptions of their administration, analysis, and interpretation, but more importantly have included in Appendix A how to obtain these measures or contact their authors in order to gain further opportunities to build expertise and competence in these techniques. For those readers who have recently begun the study of personality or have just finished a course of study in this area, this book provides a concrete demonstration of several contemporary personality theories and methods applied to the same individual, providing clear examples of how they compare and contrast with each other.

This book is by no means a comprehensive account of all facets of personality. It does not address the important contemporary advances in longitudinal and developmental personality research (Caspi & Roberts, 1999; Robins, Fraley, Roberts, & Trzesniewski, 2001), the growing field of evolutionary personality psychology (Buss, 1995; Gangestad & Simpson, 2000), or the emerging findings on implicit knowledge and the cognitive unconscious (Banaji, 2001; Bargh, 1997; Kihlstrom, 1987). Although all of these areas are yielding significant contributions to our understanding of the development and dynamics of personality, their application to a person-based therapy is a little more distant than the domains of personality research that I have chosen to highlight in this book. On the one hand, for those readers who want a more complete survey of all of personality research, I refer them to excellent current introductory textbooks by Carver and Scheier (2004) and McAdams (2006), as well as the second edition of Pervin and John's (1999) more advanced *Handbook of Personality: Theory and Research*. On the other hand, for readers who want less discussion of laboratory research in personality and more focus on the direct clinical assessment of personality and its connection to psychopathology, I recommend recent books by Beutler and Groth-Marnat (2003), Butcher (2002), and Wiggins (2003), as well as Millon and colleagues' (Millon, Davis, & Millon, 1997) influential and comprehensive body of work.

Because this book seeks to redress gaps in psychotherapists' understanding and application of contemporary personality psychology, I am also acutely aware of personality psychologists' lack of familiarity with developments in contemporary psychodynamic therapy. Due to their objectivist and empirical orientation, not to mention the subjective excesses of classical psychoanalysis, most personality psychologists have tended to give little attention to the theoretical writings and case presentations of contemporary psychoanalysts. I contend in this volume that this dismissal is a case of "throwing out the baby with the bathwater." In fact, the emerging field of relational psychoanalysis offers critical insights into a comprehensive and meaningful understanding of what it means to be (and to study) a person. Once again, one can benefit from these insights without needing to embrace the full conceptual structure and techniques of psychoanalytic therapy (I would certainly not characterize the work I do as a therapist as primarily psychoanalytic).

By synthesizing contributions from laboratory-based personality research and relational psychoanalysis, I recognize that I take the risk of all integrative efforts: I may please neither researchers nor therapists. However, in the true spirit of personality psychology's founding fathers, Gordon Allport (1937) and Henry Murray (1938), and their multidisciplinary "explorations of personality," I can see no other way of depicting in both a scientific and comprehensive manner the complexity of the whole person. Acknowledging the perils of any new endeavor, I now describe the personality-based framework that I use to understand and work with the person in psychotherapy.

THE THREE-DOMAIN
FRAMEWORK OF PERSONALITY

In the mid-1990s, Dan McAdams and Robert Emmons, two prominent personality psychologists, surveyed the field of personality and saw a fragmented but resurgent branch of psychology. Though the influence of grand theorists, whether Freud, Jung, Adler, or Skinner, had faded, advances in trait psychology, social cognition, emotion, interpersonal perspectives, and narrative psychology were reinvigorating the study of personality (see McAdams, 1997, for a history of eras and movements in 20th-century personality psychology). These positive developments, which were making their way piecemeal into revised editions of personality textbooks, led to a call by McAdams and Emmons, in a special issue of the *Journal of Personality* (December 1995, Volume 63), for a new framework of personality research that would help to organize the expanding field. Such a framework would not only allow teachers and students to convey a more relevant and accessible picture of what actually was happening in the personality research laboratories in this country and around the world, but it would also allow researchers to make connections and see opportunities for integration across different subfields of personality.

McAdams himself proposed one such framework, comprising three basic domains (McAdams, 1995, 1996), that has subsequently exerted a great influence on the field. In introducing his three-domain framework of personality research, McAdams (1995) asked his fellow personality researchers, "What Do We Know When We Know a Person?" His goal in addressing this question to the field of personality psychology was to suggest that the various investigations of personality that were mushrooming at the time could be organized around a unified framework. Using the example of an encounter at a causal evening get-together, McAdams imagined attending a party where he meets a complicated and rather strongly opinionated woman. McAdams suggested that to begin to know this person, one starts with an analysis of her traits, then moves on to consideration of her more contextualized behavior, and finally attempts to assemble from the facts of her life a more cohesive story or narrative depiction. In order to illustrate this framework, which I apply throughout this volume, let us proceed through a similar survey of McAdams's three domains with the purpose of getting to know a psychotherapy patient named Nell. Nell is an amalgam of several actual patients that I have seen over the past 20 years. Her concerns and conflicts express some of the more familiar and central themes raised by patients in my practice, but her profile is not traceable to any specific individual. I introduce Nell briefly here, but return to her in much more depth in Chapter 5, when I examine the role of relational psychotherapy in understanding the whole person.

MEETING NELL

Nell, a married woman in her early 30s, enters my office for her morning appointment. A few months back, in our first meeting, she had described a frightening mood that would overtake her late at night or in the afternoon when her young daughter was napping and her husband was at work. A gray despair would seep through her body, leaving her momentarily paralyzed, as if to move from her chair to the bedside of her sleeping child would be to climb from the bottom of a cratered beach with nothing but sheer cliffs on all sides. In some minutes, a half-hour at most, this tide of dread and sorrow would withdraw, but its memory would linger, and Nell would feel her mind and heart huddled inside her, waiting in the days to come for the next change in the air, the slight thickening of the atmosphere inside her psyche that signaled another wave ahead.

I have spent these early meetings of therapy getting to know Nell, getting used to her way of settling into my couch, how she lets her shoes fall off and curls up her knees to her chin, leaning against the armrest, as she fills me on her week. Her light scent of tea rose is now familiar, as is the way her voice fades to a near whisper when she speaks of difficult topics—her overbearing father and the strictness of her early upbringing or her ambivalence about beginning work again after time off with her child.

Though Nell has described herself as shy, she is very open with me; she often meets my eyes with directness and warmth. She is diligent about our meetings, never misses an appointment, and arrives with time to spare. In these weeks of listening to her, of asking questions to learn more about her past, her current difficulties, and her hopes for the future, I have slowly accumulated a sense of her life—how she understands and assembles its parts into a more or less cohesive story. This life narrative emphasizes her strong sense of responsibility, but a contrasting desire for self-expression. She studied art in college and has even brought some sketches and watercolors to show me. The idea of calling herself an "artist" feels too grand for her at the moment, but Nell wonders if she might find work in graphic art or book design. She has told me how she loves books, even at their most physical level—the arch of their spines or the feel of the page under her thumb. At such moments, I sense how much emotion there is beneath her reserve. Our work together in therapy thus far has returned increasingly to questions about what step Nell might take in her life to pursue her self-expression, and what such a step might mean for her marriage, her child, and her sense of identity.

Given this brief sketch, how might we begin to assemble a systematic portrait of Nell through the three-domain framework of a person-based personality psychology?

Domain 1—Traits

Traits can be defined as "dimensions of individual differences" in thoughts, feelings, and behaviors that show reasonably consistent patterns across situation, time, and role (McCrae & Costa, 2003, p. 25).

When we first meet or describe a person, traits are the most likely tools we possess to make distinctions among individuals. Nell describes herself as shy, and despite her soft-spoken nature, she conveys a sense of warmth and openness in her interactions with me. She seems to strive to please the important figures in her life—her father, her husband, and now perhaps me. The language she uses to talk about her feelings and her interest in art conveys a strong sense of imagination, a sensitivity to her own emotions, and a cultivated aesthetic sense. All of these descriptive phrases locate characteristics of Nell on dimensions of emotion and action that can be compared to other individuals on a continuum.

Trait psychology traditionally starts from these basic, common language efforts to describe people, then looks for the underlying assumptions or dimensions that would allow one to see the most fundamental linkages among the trait words used. Often, trait psychologists have assumed that these most basic trait dimensions have biological and genetic links (Eysenck, 1990; McCrae & Costa, 2003), and recent evidence from twin studies has indicated that 40 to 50% of the variance in trait scores may be linked to genetic determinants (Bouchard, Lykken, McGue, Segal, & Tellegen, 1990; Loehlin, McCrae, Costa, & John, 1998; Riemann, Angleitner, & Strelau, 1997).

The most widely used current trait measure, the Revised NEO Personality Inventory (NEO PI-R; Costa & McCrae, 1992) measures five fundamental trait dimensions: Neuroticism (management of negative emotion), Extraversion (a blend of positive emotion and activity), Openness to Experience (imagination, introspection, fantasy, flexibility about ideas and values), Agreeableness (a tendency to be compliant, trusting, tender, modest), and Conscientiousness (competence, self-discipline, achievement, orderliness). If I were to administer the NEO PI-R to Nell, I would be likely to find that she shows high levels of Openness, along with high levels of Agreeableness, while her scores on Extraversion and Conscientiousness might be more moderate. Given her proneness to bouts of sadness and anxiety, she would score moderately high on Neuroticism as well.

Individuals can vary widely in each of these five dimensions (e.g., individuals who score very high in Agreeableness are naively trusting, while those who score very low in Agreeableness are manipulative and suspicious of others), and the combination of these variations can yield a complicated and rich profile of their overall pattern of thoughts, feelings, and actions (Piedmont, 1998). Measurement of the five factors and their accompanying facets allows us to predict individuals' behavior, particularly if those predictions are based on multiple observations and not on a single encounter (Epstein, 1984). For example, having observed Nell over several weeks in meetings with her, I might indeed be able to apply the label of "agreeable" to her and show very respectable success in predicting her behavior in similar, one-on-one encounters that she has. I might also be able to predict that her friends would characterize her as a warm and gentle person in her interactions with them. I have much more to say about these "five factors" in Chapter 2, but for now, it is enough to say that these fundamental dimensions of how Nell responds to the external world, her own emotional life, and her interactions with others constitute a fundamental way of finding out who Nell is.

Domain 2—Characteristic Adaptations

Yet McAdams (1995, 1996) prompts us to ask, "Is this all we can know about a person?" Are there other features of Nell's personality that elude this trait analysis but would contribute to our understanding of her? McAdams (1995, p. 376) argued that *the* greatest strengths of traits are also their most powerful limitations: They are "comparative" and "nonconditional." First, by assigning Nell the trait of Agreeableness, I am locating her on a continuum with other individuals who share greater and lesser amounts of this characteristic. But the more I come to know about Nell, the less concerned I am with how she compares to other people. I want to know the nature of her own personal brand of Agreeableness—how she develops trusting relationships or complies with requests, even at the expense of her own well-being or needs. Increasingly, I am interested in the nature of "Agreeableness" within her and not how my initial observations of her trust or compliance match Nell to others with these characteristics.

Second, it was initially helpful for me to see Nell as agreeable across a variety of situations. She describes herself as never challenging her father and being willing to put her career goals on hold after the birth of her child, while her husband returned to work. She comes dutifully each week, and on time, to her appointments and seldom challenges my comments. In these respects, her agreeableness is "nonconditional," or consistent across a number of situations. Yet as I learn more about her in early sessions, I find out that she had periods in her high school years when she hung out with a "biker" crowd that seldom attended school and often crossed paths with the law. I also learn that she had narrowly escaped a sexual assault during these years, and that she went through a period of refusing contact with men, as well as engaging in excessive drinking and drug use. Registering Nell's initial agreeableness tells me perhaps about her primary way of organizing her interpersonal interactions, but it may not tell me about other, more conditional and contextual reactions that she may have in response to authority or to men in general. Similarly, knowing that she displays a strong aesthetic sense does not tell me anything about what this type of behavior means to her or what she might hope to achieve through expressing her artistic interests. Is she seeking freedom from interpersonal constraints, sublimating her sensuous impulses, connecting to a higher spiritual sense or aesthetic ethos, simply fighting off a sense of boredom, or responding to some combination of all these motives?

In other words, I want to know what Nell is trying to accomplish by her specific behaviors and emotional displays. I want to know what she needs, values, and seeks to avoid in specific *situations* and at certain *times* in her life, as well as in the particular *roles* she occupies in her relationships with others. How was her artistic impulse expressed when she was 10 years younger, and how might she hope to express it 10 years hence? I want to know whether she feels these desires when she is at home with her husband, out with her friends, or on a walk with her child. Each of these moments for Nell may reflect a different "self-with-other" representation or role relationship (Horowitz, 1991; Ogilvie, Fleming, & Pennell, 1998), and all of these combined moments may approach a more accurate picture of Nell's whole person than a nonconditional trait analysis. Finally, what does she hide from others and from me in order to protect herself against anxieties and fears related to her desires and goals? How does she adopt coping strategies and defensive styles to disguise feelings or thoughts that might make her appear vulnerable to others and to herself?

Asking these questions, according to McAdams, enables us to learn about how Nell generates *characteristic adaptations* that fit her personality to the demands of time, situation, and role. As Henry Murray (1938) pointed out long ago, human beings experience needs that are energized into motives by interactions with *presses* or cues from the environment. Characteristic adaptations are the reasonably stable confluences of needs and contexts in our lives.

Domain 3—Narrative Identity and Meaning Making

The third domain of McAdams's framework concerns how Nell finds meaning in her needs and their role in her life. Contemporary society requires that individuals respond in a unique and personal way to the questions "Who are you?" and "What does your life mean?" For much of history, such questions could be answered by recourse to one's membership in a particular family, religious community, social class, or vocational role (Baumeister, 1986). Since the advent of sweeping economic, cultural, spiritual, and technological changes that gained momentum in the 19th century and accelerated in the 20th century to reach the dizzying pace of our 21st-century society, to answer these two questions individuals have increasingly needed to rely on their own efforts at self-definition and meaning-making rather than drawing on external structures of family, class, or faith. As contemporary society divides and fragments our lives into disparate spheres and functions that may change multiple times in our own lifetimes due to technological advances, the need for a sense of unity and purpose in our own lives is greater than ever.

McAdams (1995) proposed that the construction of *identity* (Erikson, 1963) is the task of bringing unity and purpose to the self across the life course. Identity is the psychosocial construct that meaningfully locates us in a sociocultural niche and unifies our lives temporally by finding continuity among our previous experiences, present concerns, and future aspirations. For contemporary individuals, identity construction is accomplished through the crafting of an ongoing *life story*. In other words, beginning in adolescence, individuals start to assemble the events of their lives into a narrative that connects past, present, and anticipated future. The ongoing work on a coherent life story provides direction and purpose in their lives, while simultaneously linking them to the dominant stories of their society and culture.

This third domain of understanding or describing Nell, then, concerns how Nell herself constructs a narrative of her life—how she tells the story of who she is, and what meanings she assigns to this story. In my meetings with Nell thus far, I have taken in many elements of this story. Part of my work as a therapist is to collect an extensive history, and my history taking usually extends over several sessions. From these initial efforts (and there are always more elements to the life story that are added or modified over time), I know Nell sees herself engaged in a struggle to assert her autonomy in the face of authoritarian men and traditional society. I know she also loves the gentleness that has characterized many of her relationships and that has been expressed with a depth that even Nell had not expected in her care for her daughter. I know she sees the episodes of rebellion in high school and college not only as periods of desperate acting out but also as reminders of a defiant streak in herself that she cannot suppress. I know she sees her recent bouts of depression as a warning to herself that she feels trapped again in a role that does not allow her more expressive and exuberant aspects to emerge. Nell has woven all of this information into the life-history account that she has given of herself.

These themes and insights are also linked to specific memories of incidents in Nell's life that underlie these ideas and reinforce their importance to her. As I explore in great depth in Chapter 5, Nell at one point provides a memory from her teenage years of going for a hike, standing on a mountainside, and then becoming lost temporarily. We will see in fact how this self-defining memory captures the perfect blending of past experience and the themes and conflicts that shape Nell's ongoing self-concept. The connections she makes between the past events of her life and her current conflicts and desires are most definitely the stuff of McAdams's Domain 3—Identity and Meaning Making.

MISSING ELEMENTS

McAdams (1995) finished his discussion by asking what is missing? First, the framework neither explains why a person shows the characteristics of each of the domains nor how the domains might account for each other. In McAdams's language, it is a descriptive, not an explanatory model—a framework and not a theory of personality.

Second, and highly relevant to psychotherapy, is the issue of how conscious or unconscious these elements of the person might be. McAdams (1995) suggested that all three domains exist along a "gradient of consciousness" (p. 389). In other words, individuals can have relative degrees of awareness of any of the constructs located at each of the three domains. Nell is indeed highly aware of her tendency to be agreeable and sometimes takes action about this trait. She is also aware of her striving to gain more opportunity for artistic expression. However, she may be much less aware of a conflicting striving to avoid failure or embarrassment if her efforts at autonomy were not to succeed. She may see others as preventing her expressing herself but be less aware of her own contribution to holding back her self-expression. Clearly, Nell shows much awareness about major themes that organize her life story at Domain 3, but does she know fully where her child fits into this life story? For example, is it possible that her bouts of paralysis when her child sleeps might reflect unconscious wishes not to come to her child's aid or to check on her well-being? Would Nell, who perceives herself as a gentle and loving person (quite accurately, in my opinion), allow into her life story the fantasy of abandoning or removing her child from the world? These questions suggest that to know Nell fully as a person, I need to draw on theory and research that helps me understand the role of conscious and *unconscious* processes in her personality—how awareness and a lack of awareness combine to influence her affect, behavior, goals, and meaning making.

With these additions then, do we have a working framework that will allow us to find the person, the individual who enters either the research laboratory or the therapy office? McAdams's framework, in its elegance and comprehensiveness, has brought us a long way. It is a powerful way to organize my understanding of the people with whom I work in psychotherapy and, as we have already seen, it allows for description of many critical aspects of Nell. In subsequen rely on it extensively to build my picture of the whole-persu.. tive. In Chapters 2, 3, and 4, it forms the basis of my exposition of personality psychology's efforts to describe the person. Yet, to return to McAdams's persistent question, "What else is missing?"

THE FOURTH DOMAIN OF RELATIONAL DYNAMICS

Thorne and Latzke (1996), in responding to McAdams's framework, cautioned that it does not fully take into account the relational context of its three domains.

> Life stories, as well as traits and [characteristic adaptations], are co-constructed implicitly or explicitly with other people. We learn about our abilities and our identities by being pestered with questions about who we are from other people, by presenting ourselves to other people, by negotiating our identity with that of others. . . . Hunkering down with persons as they tell their life stories and being sensitive to the ways in which we reciprocally influence the telling of life stories is a highly productive way to understand the process of [constructing the self]. To whom and for whom does the I construct the Me? Are the I and the Me enough? Must not we also include the You? (p. 375)

These words seem to me particularly apt in the context of memories and life stories expressed in the course of psychotherapy. As psychoanalysts interested in narrative have claimed (Schafer, 1983; Spence, 1982), a "narrative truth" may emerge from the co-constructive work of patient and therapist that cannot be mapped perfectly into the veridical past experiences of the patient. The story that emerges, which provides a meaningful and healing structure to the reconstructive efforts of the patient, invariably bears the stamp of the values, feelings, and past experiences of the therapist. Even more though, there is something called "intersubjectivity"—a world or space created that belongs to neither the patient's nor the therapist's past (Stolorow & Atwood, 1992). This transactional reality, which is different from Nell's or the therapist's internal self-with-other representation, is what Ogden (1994) calls "the analytic third."

To know about Nell, I need to recognize how my knowledge includes what happens when my knowing her fuses with her knowing me. The coming together of our traits, characteristic adaptations, memories, and life stories creates a third self-with-other entity that exists neither within Nell nor within me. What might this intersubjective awareness mean for my understanding of Nell?

Two points are relevant to this question. First, I am learning about how Nell forms relationships—how she is experienced by another person and how she experiences me. I am learning this not simply through her self-report, but through a real-time transaction that engages my entire personality—feelings, thoughts, bodily sensations. I am also learning about what Nell may not be able to put into words and to experience consciously within herself.

Melanie Klein (1975) originated the term "projective identification," and Ogden (1991) has written extensively about this process, particularly with regard to more disturbed patients. In brief, projective identification is the process whereby the patient unconsciously creates a feeling in the therapist that is unacceptable or intolerable to hold within the patient's own self. The therapist then experiences this feeling as his or her own feeling. Through reflection, and often with the aid of a colleague or supervisor, the therapist may be lucky enough to identify this feeling (usually rage, shame, or fear) as a projection from the patient. Whether or not the therapist is able to recognize what is happening, the patient's psyche is carefully monitoring and "identifying" with what the therapist does with this feeling. Ideally, the therapist is able to model an acceptable response and tolerance of this split-off part of the patient. By demonstrating to the patient that the incorporation of such frightening impulses into the self is not toxic or destructive of the self, the therapist provides the patient with an increased capacity for tolerating these feelings and self-acceptance.

To know about Nell most fully, I need to register and make sense of potential projective identifications that take place in our mutual, ongoing self-with-other transactions. In Chapter 5, I explore these processes in much more depth as I pursue what relational psychoanalysis has to teach about the full extent of the person in relationship that might not be revealed by more traditional personality measurement, not even those forms of assessment that examine interpersonal patterns in therapy (e.g., Crits-Christoph, Demorest, Muenz, & Baranackie, 1994; Horowitz, 1991; Kiesler, 2002; Knapp, 1991; Luborsky & Crits-Christoph, 1998).

I should note here though that while relational psychotherapy is a vehicle for identifying this intersubjective world shared by individuals, this dimension of human nature is by no means limited to psychotherapy. In all human interactions, and particularly in our most intimate ones, we inhabit shared subjective worlds that allow for communication in symbolic and often unconscious manners. To know or understand individuals fully means taking into account these shifting relational dynamics. Ultimately, a science of the person that seeks to treat the person as an isolated entity, extracted from these relational influences, is likely to be an incomplete enterprise.

When modern psychology evolved as its own discipline in the 19th century, it ultimately accepted a positivist stance toward the study of human beings, adopting as its model the principles and methods of the natural sciences and physics. However, as I argue in this volume, personality psychology, as conceptualized by Allport (1937), has additional roots in a second tradition that also emerged at the end of the 19th century and that questioned the appropriateness of this disengaged position in the study of human beings. The German phenomenologist Wilhelm Dilthey (1894/1977) argued that there are indeed two discrete activities in our efforts to understand the world. He called the familiar positivist approach *erklären* science, or the effort to explain the world in more objective and naturalistic terms. In contemporary personality psychology, this approach translates into the use of questionnaires, experimental studies, and statistical techniques, such as scaling, factor analysis, and analysis of variance.

In contrast, there is *verstehen* psychology, or the effort to understand human beings in their own context and to make sense of the subjective meanings they construct of their life experience. *Verstehen* psychology requires the use of hermeneutic and interpretive methods that focus on a sensitivity to and exploration of symbols, metaphors, and cultural influences in the lives of the people we study and treat. With the advances of feminist and narrative approaches across many disciplines of psychology, there has indeed been a resurgence of interest in and respect for this *verstehen* approach. A personality psychology, which seeks to describe the whole person through an account of his or her traits, characteristic adaptations, and life stories, also needs to depict individuals in the midst of the phenomenological worlds they inhabit. To accomplish this goal, I shall at times, and with caution, draw on interpretive methods that let go of the disengaged stance of *erklären* science. To do so is not to veer away from the science of personality, but to regain the original spirit and intent with which Allport fashioned personality psychology.

In the chapters ahead, I systematically build this framework that leads to the treatment of the whole person. To do so, I need to leave Nell temporarily in order to construct a step-by-step empirical account of another individual (in this case an actual research volunteer with the pseudonym "Jennifer"), based in the methods of personality psychology. I then return to Nell to illustrate the application of more interpretive methods, based in relational psychotherapy. Finally, in the last chapter of this volume, I bring the techniques of the laboratory and the clinic together by presenting a case study of couples treatment that draws on all four domains of a person-based personality psychology. In the remainder of this chapter, let us take a brief look at each of the subsequent chapters.

THE CHAPTERS AHEAD

Chapters 2, 3 and 4 present a sample of measures from each domain of McAdams's framework. My assumption in these chapters is that all of the measures employed may be relatively new to the reader. Each chapter presents the results from the laboratory study of Jennifer, the aforementioned volunteer research participant. This analysis from the three-domain perspective grew out of a research seminar on personality that I taught at Connecticut College. I asked the nine students in the seminar to assess a single person over the course of a 16-week semester, meeting with the person five or six times, with each meeting ranging from 30 minutes to 2 hours. Each participant to be studied in this project was a student from an Introductory Psychology course who earned experimental credit toward his or her course requirements. They received the NEO PI-R (Domain 1), a measure of personal strivings (long-term goals), a measure of adjustment and defensiveness (Domain 2), a life-history interview, and a self-defining memory task (Domain 3). The students in my seminar and I then worked together as a group and in independent meetings to develop an integrative whole-person analysis of each individual. In some ways, my goal was to replicate the collaborative study of a person exemplified by Henry Murray's (1938) diagnostic council.

The outcome was a final report that not only captured the person at each of McAdams's three domains but also sought to make connections across the domains (for a parallel example, see McAdams's analysis of Madeleine G. in Wiggins, 2003). I selected "Jennifer's" profile to provide an accessible introduction to how one can conduct an analysis at each domain and then bring the domains together to make an integrative description out of these results. Even for clinicians long removed from courses in personality psychology, my discussion of the measures and analyses involved is at a level that should be user-friendly and straightforward in its application of the personality instruments.

In Chapter 5, I step away from the laboratory and ask what we might learn about a person from applying a subjective, engaged, interpretive approach in contrast to the detached and objective stance taken thus far. My interpretive approach returns to Nell and an examination of knowledge gained through the therapeutic relationship. The chapter traces the historical emergence of the major themes of relational psychoanalysis and explores their relevance to the person-based personality psychology that I have been developing in the previous three chapters. In particular, I place a special focus on a memory Nell recounts and show how it reflects both her own life struggles and the relationships she forms with others (including her therapeutic relationship).

In summary then, the combination of Chapters 2–4 and Chapter 5 should provide complementary takes on what constitutes a person-based perspective. Chapters 2–4 not only work from a more laboratory-based research approach but also provide clear examples of personality instruments that one might use in psychotherapy practice (once again, see Appendix A for information about websites and how to obtain each instrument). Chapter 5 builds from the clinical setting rather than the laboratory, but still offers a strong sampling of theory and research on personality and interpersonal processes critical to an understanding of the individual.

These chapters combined should move us closer to an answer about how we might understand the person, but they leave two important questions for the final two chapters:

1. Given the growing influence of neuroscience and cognitive science on psychotherapy, is there still a scientific and intellectual justification for this person-based perspective in psychotherapy?
2. Assuming that there is a scientific justification for this person-based perspective, how do we apply this perspective to therapy, and what are its benefits for the people with whom we work?

Chapter 6 addresses the first of these two questions by arguing that all therapies must be accountable for how they conceptualize their understanding of a person. The methods and outcomes that characterize different therapeutic approaches ultimately reflect ethical stances about what is valued and promoted within our society. Identifying dimensions of free will and independence–interdependence as critical factors in one's vision of a person, I highlight the tendency of cognitive-behavioral and biological treatments to characterize individuals in an overly individualistic and mechanistic fashion. Such characterizations neglect the relational and sociopolitical contexts of individual lives, while simultaneously underplaying individuals' efforts toward integration and meaning making. In contrast, a person-based psychotherapy blends a humanistic concern for purpose and meaning with an awareness of the social, cultural, and relational circumstances that are unique to each individual. In place of heavily deterministic views of human nature that tend to see either biology or environmental conditioning as destiny, a person-based perspective is highly sensitive to the possibility of self-initiated change over the course of an individual's life. In Chapter 6, I state each of these premises more formally, offering a clear framework and set of principles to guide personality psychology and psychotherapy.

In Chapter 7, I turn to an actual demonstration of a person-based therapy by presenting the case study of a couple in marital distress. The case study illustrates how couples therapy can draw on the concepts and instruments of personality psychology to help each member of the couple develop greater self-understanding and understanding of his or her partner. Through application of measures of traits, characteristic adaptations, and life narratives presented in the Chapters 2–4, as well as a commitment to the relational framework laid out in Chapter 5, I am able to demonstrate both the depth of insight and the practical utility offered by a person-based psychotherapy. For clinicians interested in incorporating some of the ideas promulgated in this volume in their own practice, Chapter 7 describes exercises and clinical interventions within the couples work that help convey the essence of the person-based perspective.

After presenting the person-based case study, I conclude Chapter 7 by describing related research and clinical work that promote a similar concern with narrative and meaning making in order to understand and aid the person. Both personality and clinical literatures, not to mention developments in cognitive neuroscience as well (Baars, 2002; LeDoux, 1996), are converging on the position that the integration of different systems within the personality is a signal of optimal adjustment for the individual. Individuals who are able to combine narratives of emotional experiences with reflection and meaning making show improved physical and psychological health, as well as higher levels of maturity, wisdom, and ego development. I review evidence for this claim from diverse researchers, including James Pennbaker, Laura King, Leslie Greenberg and Lynne Angus, and Lester Luborsky, as well as the clinical case studies of Michael White and his narrative therapy approach. I offer these examples as both evidence of and encouragement for positive alternatives to economic, bureaucratic, and ostensibly "scientific" forces that depersonalize psychotherapy.

Ultimately, and most critically, psychotherapy linked to personality psychology attends to the full complexity of the individual person and that individual's efforts to find meaning and purpose in life. When Nell moves from discussion of her depression to fundamental questions about the meaning of an event in her life that took place 17 years before, she is asking for more than a short-term palliative response to her current sadness. She wants to understand why a brief episode nearly two decades earlier that ostensibly altered nothing in that day's routine or her life at that time persists in her memory and feels like one of the most self-defining moments of her life. Whatever else I do in my work as a personality psychologist and psychotherapist, it is my effort to help her answer this fascinating question that expresses the particular kind of contribution that is at the heart of treating the whole person. It is not the only form of therapy, and it is by no means the appropriate approach in all cases or with all people, but it is what a psychotherapy informed by personality psychology has to offer Nell—insight into the themes and conflicts that encompass the fullest possible picture of her humanity.

2

Domain 1—Traits

In this chapter, the first domain of personality psychology is put to work through the study of Jennifer, a 21-year-old college senior, who has reached that particular crossroads at which her entrance into the "real world" is only a few short months away. By studying her basic disposition through a trait assessment, I seek to lay a foundation for the development of an integrated picture of her personality that follows in the next two chapters. Inevitably, there is much more that we might ask and learn about Jennifer; our inquiry and analysis is too brief and incomplete. Yet my hope is that by at least sampling from each of the three domains of personality, I can make a compelling case for the importance of considering all three domains in any effort to reach a more comprehensive understanding of another person.

In setting my goal to study a single person across all three domains of personality, I inevitably had to make choices about methods of assessment at each level. Since my goal is to the lay the foundations of a person-based psychology that can be applied in clinical settings, I chose measures with the following criteria in mind: First, each measure should be scientifically researched, with evidence of reliability, validity, and successful application to questions of personality adjustment, well-being, and health.

Second, each measure should be easily administered, time-efficient, and widely used. As a clinician myself, I realize that most therapists tend not to employ formal assessment instruments in their private practices. Yet I have chosen instruments that can be incorporated into practice without requiring hours of administration time and analysis. Even more,

I have tried to choose instruments that have a valuable conceptual framework associated with them. So even if clinicians do not give clients the actual instruments, they might still benefit from keeping the critical questions raised by these measures in their minds as they work with their patients. Ultimately, if personality analyses are to have meaning and utility to full-time therapists who are constantly juggling hours of practice with clinical notes, phone calls, managed care paperwork, referral requests, legal requests, continuing education, and any ongoing writing or research, these methods must yield their information in an efficient and focused way.

Third, I chose assessment measures that are compatible with a range of psychotherapeutic orientations. The trait inventory approach for the first domain fits within an empirical and nosological paradigm of personality assessment that is favored by a medical model and DSM-IV (*Diagnostic and Statistical Manual of Mental Disorders*) perspective (Wiggins, 2003). My focus on assessment of long-term goals for the second domain fits well within both cognitive-behavioral and psychodynamic therapeutic approaches. Similarly, an additional analysis within the second domain of adjustment and defensive styles enlists an understanding of cognitive-behavioral adaptations and a psychodynamic emphasis on defensive avoidance of anxiety. Finally, the use of a life-history interview and collection of autobiographical memories cuts across all types of therapies but particularly engages a humanistic orientation toward identity formation and meaning making.

It is important to recognize that a laboratory assessment of personality (even one of several hours' duration over a number of weeks) cannot reach the same depth of understanding that a therapist achieves through weekly encounters with a patient over several months. Yet, in a sense, this limited degree of depth serves my purposes well. I do not want to forsake the forest for the trees. A major objective in studying Jennifer is to show the utility of applying these three domains to an understanding of the personality of clients in practice. By applying this framework to actual clients, the therapist can then draw on more intensive work with each person to fill in the details and complexity for each of the domains (see Chapter 7 for my own clinical example of this process).

BACKGROUND OF THE DEVELOPMENT OF THE FIVE-FACTOR PERSPECTIVE AND THE NEO PI-R

Given the importance of the "Big Five" approach in contemporary psychology, it would be helpful to see how psychologists arrived at this set of fundamental traits. In the brief history that follows, I emphasize the development of the most widely used five-factor instrument, the NEO PI-R (Costa & McCrae, 1992; McCrae & Costa, 2003). However, it should be noted that several other scientifically reliable and valid five-factor instruments and approaches are available (Digman, 1989; Goldberg, 1990; John & Srivastava, 1999).

The notion of characterizing individuals by their variation in fundamental dimensions of temperament or behavior can be traced at least as far back as 400 B.C.E., when Hippocratus proposed a typology of personality based on bodily fluids.

The Greek physician Galen revived this scheme in 150 C.E. and made the following associations of "bodily humors" to personality types. An excess of

Blood led to a "sanguine" temperament or a lively, talkative person.
Black bile led to a "melancholic" temperament or a sober, pessimistic individual.
Yellow bile led to a "choleric" temperament or an angry, impulsive individual.
Phlegm led to a "phlegmatic" temperament or a slow-to-react, mellow individual.

Since this initial nosology, various schemes of dividing up individuals by fundamental characteristics have emerged with varying popularity and persistence over the centuries, including astrological and phrenological distinctions, as well approaches based on ethnic heritage (Galton, 1884) and bodily physique (Kretschmer, 1921; Sheldon, 1940). Even the great philosopher Immanuel Kant talked about dimensions of activity and feeling, and the founder of the first psychology laboratory, Wilhelm Wundt, saw the four temperaments as based in variations of emotional strength and consistency (see McAdams, 2006).

In the mid-20th century, Allport (1937) formally defined the notion of a trait as a characteristic disposition with an underlying neural basis that tends to impose similar perceptions on diverse stimuli and that guides behavior in a rather predictable and stable direction. In an effort to develop an inductive understanding of personality traits, Allport and Odbert (1936) identified 18,000 trait-descriptive terms in the English language. The challenge then was to reduce this wealth of words into a more workable framework of personality traits. Allport and Odbert distilled the 18,000 descriptive terms to 4,000 personality-specific terms. From there, Cattell (1946) formed clusters of synonyms, eventually yielding 35 groups that he worked into a personality questionnaire. Just as one simmers chicken, vegetables, and herbs to reach the most potent

stock for soup, Cattell continued to distill his dimensions through pro-
gressive factor analyses until he reached 16 fundamental factors—the
widely used Sixteen Personality Factor Questionnaire (16PF; Cattell,
Eber, & Tatsuoka, 1970). To give examples of his factors, one might
consider some representative dimensions, which Cattell identified by letters of the alphabet: A—Worrying (high) versus Self-Assured (low);
Q1—Radical (high) versus Conservative (low); F—Cheerful (high) versus Lively (low); or E—Assertive (high) versus Humble (low).

Around the same time that Cattell was developing his 16 factors,
British psychologist Hans Eysenck (1952) was using a different form of
factor analysis to reduce the fundamental traits to an even more concen-
trated broth. Cattell's approach allowed for some overlap or correlation
among his factors; each factor represented its own dimension, but it also
shared features of some other dimensions as well. For example, Dimension A—Outgoing versus Reserved was not completely independent of
Dimension F—Cheerful versus Sober. In contrast, Eysenck set limits on
his factors that demanded that they share no overlap from one factor to
the next. This more stringent test distilled the remaining dimensions to a
fundamental three: Extraversion–Introversion, Neuroticism, and Psy-
choticism. The first dimension captures one's overall tendency to be outgoing versus reserved; the second, one's proneness to stable, positive
emotion versus restless, negative emotion; and the third, one's inclination toward asocial or antisocial behavior, including lapses with reality,
law breaking, and failures of empathy.

As Eysenck (1973, cited in McAdams, 2006) described it, one could
think of these first two dimensions as reflecting the combination of
Galen's four humors. Individuals high in extraversion and low in
neuroticism would be likely to be optimistic, energetic leaders (sanguine). Individuals low in extraversion and high in neuroticism would be
pessimistic, moody, and withdrawn (melancholic). High scores in extraversion and neuroticism would lead to a touchy, restless, and impulsive
profile (choleric), while low scores in both extraversion and neuroticism
would yield an even-tempered and rather passive individual (phlegmatic).

Eysenck (1990) conducted many studies over the years that suggest
these differences in personality might indeed be linked to a tolerance for
arousal. Individuals who are introverted may have a very high baseline
of arousal; they need little to get them excited or stimulated. In contrast,
extraverts may have a low baseline and require much more stimulation
to move from a calm to an aroused state. This theory has successfully
predicted many differences between the two kinds of individuals. For example, introverted individuals can drink more alcohol before showing
any effects (they start at a high level of arousal and require more of the

depressant effect of alcohol to become affected). Extraverted individuals, on the other hand, start at a lower level of arousal and respond more immediately to the depressant influence of alcohol on their bodies. It is the exact opposite for a stimulant drug like cocaine; introverts need much less and extraverts, much more.

For a while, it seemed like Eysenck's three "supertraits" would carry the day, but other researchers periodically found additional dimensions that did not quite fall neatly into this triad. Using Cattell's 35 rating scales, two researchers, Tupes and Christal (1961), carried out a series of investigations that yielded not Cattell's 16 or Eysenck's three, but five fundamental dimensions. Norman (1963) replicated their findings, and almost 20 years later, Goldberg (1981, 1982), working from his own set of dictionary-generated synonyms, again obtained five dimensions. Norman had labeled these factors Extraversion or Surgency, Agreeableness, Conscientiousness, Emotional Stability, and Culture. Agreeableness expressed individuals' tendency to seek acceptance from others and to be conciliatory, trusting, tender, and compliant. Conscientiousness encompassed aspects of competence, dutifulness, achievement, and self-discipline, while Culture tapped into individuals' interest in matters of intellect, aesthetics, and imagination.

In the mid-1970s, Paul Costa and Robert R. "Jeff" McCrae (1976) were engaged in a research project sponsored by the Boston Veteran Administration to study aging longitudinally. Though they began with the 16PF, their own factor analysis of their sample results yielded three prominent factors: Two matched Eysenck's Neuroticism and Extraversion, but the third defined a different construct that reflected one's proneness to imagination and aesthetic experiences—a kind of flexibility in moving between one's internal thoughts and the experiences of the external world. They called this dimension Openness to Experience. Working with their three factors, they developed the NEO PI, measuring dimensions of Neuroticism, Extraversion, and Openness to Experience. However, by the early 1980s, they learned of Goldberg's (1981, 1982) progress and his confirmation of the earlier work by Tupes and Christal (1961), as well as Norman (1963).

Adding Agreeableness and Conscientiousness to their three factors, McCrae and Costa (1985, 1989, 1990; Costa & McCrae, 1992) proceeded to validate this five-factor model (FFM) in a large adult sample of men and women as a part of the Baltimore Longitudinal Study of Aging, utilizing the revised version of their original instrument, now called the Revised NEO Personality Inventory (NEO PI-R). As documented in McCrae and Costa (1999), they subsequently recovered their five factors of Neuroticism (N), Extraversion (E), Openness (O), Agreeableness (A), and Conscientiousness (C) in self-reports on adjective lists (Saucier,

1997), expert ratings of personality (Lanning, 1994), questionnaires measuring needs and motives (Costa & McCrae, 1988), and symptom clusters of personality disorders (Clark & Livesley, 1994). Their identification of the five factors has extended to cross-cultural studies (McCrae, Costa, et al., 1998; McCrae et al., 1999) and applications to the workplace (Barrick & Mount, 1991). Additionally, five-factor researchers are increasingly accumulating evidence that these dimensions are heritable, in other words, that they have a genetic origin (Loehlin et al., 1998; Riemann et al., 1997).

In recent theoretical statements, McCrae and Costa (1999, 2003) have proposed a five-factor theory of personality that places the five factors as the biological base of personality or "basic tendencies" from which more contextual adaptations and the self-concept are derived (see Figure 2.1); that is, we begin life with biotemperamental inclinations toward Extraversion, Neuroticism, Openness to Experience, Agreeableness, and Conscientiousness. The interaction of these emotional and behavioral proclivities with our social environment yields characteristic patterns of responding to the world, as well as internal self-schemas and self-representations. Though Goldberg (Saucier & Goldberg, 1996), one of the original five-factor proponents, has cautioned about the rush to biological causal explanations, Buss (1996) has suggested linkages of the five factors to "difference-detecting mechanisms" that might have been evolutionary adaptations to aid in survival and reproduction (John & Srivastava, 1999). Gosling (Gosling & John, 1999) has also begun a program of research that explores affective–behavioral correlates of the five factors in nonhuman animals.

The convergence of researchers around the FFM has led to a renewed enthusiasm for the trait perspective in not only personality psychology but also clinical psychology. As documented by Costa and Widiger (2002), numerous clinical and personality psychologists have begun to explore the mapping of the five factors onto diagnostic categories from the DSM-IV-R, as well as the utility of the NEO PI-R for clinical assessment and treatment guidance (e.g., Piedmont, 1998).

DESCRIPTION AND ADMINISTRATION OF THE NEO PI-R

Table 2.1 displays the big five dimensions and the underlying six facets associated with each dimension. If we reconfigure the order of the factors, we can create the acronym OCEAN as a mnemonic to remember all five. There are 240 items in the NEO PI-R, eight items for each of the six facets for each of the five dimensions ($8 \times 6 \times 5 = 240$). The items are

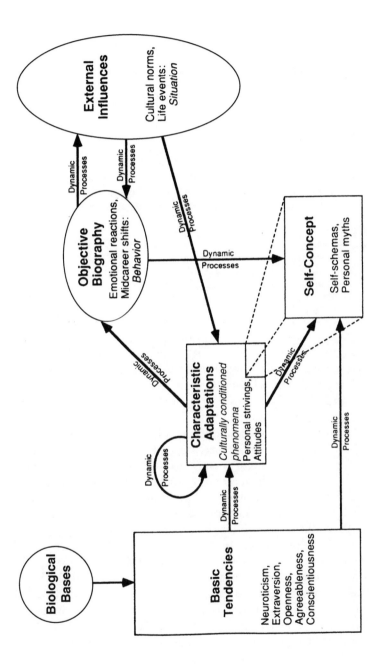

FIGURE 2.1. A representation of the five-factor theory personality system. Core components are in rectangles; interfacing components are in ellipses. From McCrae and Costa (2003, p. 92). Copyright 2003 by The Guilford Press. Reprinted by permission.

TABLE 2.1. The Five Factors and Their Facets

Neuroticism	Agreeableness
(N1—Anxiety)	(A1—Trust)
(N2 Angry Hostility)	(A2—Straightforwardness)
(N3—Depression)	(A3—Altruism)
(N4—Self-Consciousness)	(A4—Compliance)
(N5—Impulsiveness)	(A5—Modesty)
(N6—Vulnerability)	(A6—Tender-Minded)
Extraversion	Conscientiousness
(E1—Warmth)	(C1—Competence)
(E2—Gregariousness)	(C2—Order)
(E3—Assertiveness)	(C3—Dutifulness)
(E4—Activity)	(C4—Achievement Striving)
(E5—Excitement Seeking)	(C5—Self-Discipline)
(E6—Positive Emotions)	(C6—Deliberation)
Openness	
(O1—Fantasy)	
(O2—Aesthetics)	
(O3—Feelings)	
(O4—Actions)	
(O5—Ideas)	
(O6—Values)	

arranged on a 5-point scale with *strongly disagree* and *strongly agree* at the extreme anchors. The NEO PI-R comes in two versions—Form S for self-reports and Form R for observer ratings (usually made by a peer, partner, or expert); it is also available in a form for adolescents and young adults, as well as in the adult version. There is a short form of the inventory, the NEO Five-Factor Inventory, a 60-item version that is scored for the five domains only. I chose to use the extended NEO PI-R in order to have access to the facet scores and the additional interpretive information they provide. For more information about obtaining copies of the inventory, as well as computer-administered and scored versions, please see Appendix A, this volume.

To give you a flavor of the items for each of the five dimensions, I have provided some sample items for each dimension along with the facet that it measures in parentheses after the item (Table 2.2). It should be noted that there are reversed items for each facet. For example, N1 (Anxiety) has the reversed item, "I am not a worrier"; O3 (Feelings) has the reversed item, "I seldom pay much attention to my feelings of the moment," and C4 (Achievement Striving) has the reversed item, "I don't feel like I'm driven to get ahead."

TABLE 2.2. Sample Items for the Facets of the NEO PI-R

Neuroticism
I often feel tense and jittery. (N1—Anxiety)
I often get angry at the way people treat me. (N2 Angry Hostility)
Sometimes I feel completely worthless. (N3—Depression)
In dealing with other people, I always dread making a social blunder.
    (N4—Self-Consciousness)
I have trouble resisting my cravings. (N5—Impulsiveness)
I often feel helpless and want someone else to solve my problems.
    (N6—Vulnerability)

Extraversion
I really like most people I meet. (E1—Warmth)
I like to have a lot of people around me. (E2—Gregariousness)
I am dominant, forceful, and assertive. (E3—Assertiveness)
When I do things, I do them vigorously. (E4—Activity)
I often crave excitement. (E5—Excitement-Seeking)
I am a cheerful high-spirited person. (E6—Positive Emotions)

Openness
I have a very active imagination. (O1—Fantasy)
I am intrigued by patterns I find in art and nature. (O2—Aesthetics)
I experience a wide range of feelings and emotions. (O3—Feelings)
I often try new and foreign foods. (O4—Actions)
I have a lot of intellectual curiosity. (O5—Ideas)
I consider myself broad-minded and tolerant of other people's lifestyles.
    (O6—Values)

Agreeableness
I believe that most of the people I deal with are honest and trustworthy.
    (A1—Trust)
I am not crafty or sly. (A2—Straightforwardness)
I try to be courteous to everyone I meet. (A3—Altruism)
I would rather cooperate with others than compete. (A4—Compliance)
I try to be humble. (A5—Modesty)
Political leaders need to be more aware of the human side of their policies.
    (A6—Tender-Minded)

Conscientiousness
I am efficient and effective at work. (C1—Competence)
I keep my belongings neat and clean. (C2—Order)
When I make a commitment, I can always be counted on to follow through.
    (C3—Dutifulness)
I strive for excellence in everything I do. (C4—Achievement Striving)
Once I start a project, I almost always finish it. (C5—Self-Discipline)
I always consider the consequences before I take action. (C6—Deliberation)

The hand-scored version of the NEO PI-R is presented in a booklet form, and the individual fills out an accompanying bubble answer sheet. Most respondents take between 30 and 40 minutes to complete the inventory. Jennifer filled out the NEO PI-R Form S in approximately 30 minutes. Before reporting the results of Jennifer's scores, let us learn some of her most basic demographic details.

DEMOGRAPHIC BACKGROUND OF JENNIFER

Jennifer, a 21-year-old college senior at a highly selective, private liberal arts college, comes from an upper-middle-class suburban community in New England. Her older brother attends the same college with her. She was raised in the Catholic faith, but indicates that her family was not particularly religious. She plays an intercollegiate sport and has a long history of athletic activity, dating back to extensive training and competition as a figure skater prior to high school. She transferred to her current college after attending a small university in the Mid-Atlantic region for the first 2 years. She has chosen a Humanities major and performs in the B+ range for most of her subjects.

One other striking detail about Jennifer is her physical appearance. She is unusually beautiful, according to the conventions of almost any contemporary culture. In other words, she is tall; athletically trim; and has long, straight, dark hair and highly symmetrical features. She dresses in modest, almost conservative attire but is clearly meticulous about her appearance. I will have occasion to go into much greater detail about her life history in subsequent chapters, but it is helpful to have the basic outline of Jennifer in mind as we begin to fill in the different domains of her personality.

SCORING OF THE NEO PI-R

There are three validity statements at the end of the NEO PI-R concerning whether the respondent answered all items, put responses in the correct boxes, and responded honestly and accurately. Jennifer answered positively to these queries and therefore produced a valid profile. Additionally, she showed enough variation in both her overall agreement and disagreement with items that there was no evidence of either an acquiescing or nay-saying response style (Costa & McCrae, 1992, p. 6).

To obtain Jennifer's scores for each facet and for each dimension, I totaled her eight items for each facet, and then added the six facet scores together to create a raw score for each of the five dimensions. The facet scores and each dimension's raw total may then be plotted on a profile form, which converts the raw scores to T-scores, with a mean of 50 and a standard deviation of 10. The T-scores are based on various normative samples. High scores are in the 55–65 range; very high scores are in the 65–80 range; average scores are in the 45–55 range; low scores are in the 35–45 range; and very low scores are in the 20–35 range. In Jennifer's case, we used the female college-age sample form to generate her profile (though this form is for a 17–20 age group, Jennifer had only recently turned 21 and was still enrolled in college).

Figure 2.2 displays Jennifer's profile for the five dimensions and each of the 30 facets.

INTERPRETING JENNIFER'S PROFILE

To begin to make sense of a NEO PI-R profile, we start with the five broad domain scores. As Figure 2.2 indicates, Jennifer's highest score was 66 in Agreeableness (very high), which placed her 1.6 standard deviations above average in this domain. Agreeableness is a domain that measures interpersonal tendencies to get along with others and to show sympathy and altruistic concern. High scorers are eager to please others, highly trusting, and eager to avoid conflict. However, Costa and McCrae (1990, 1992) found that very high scores are associated with a tendency toward dependent personality disorder. The features of this disorder include difficulty making everyday decisions without an excessive amount of advice and reassurance from others; difficulty expressing disagreement with others; difficulty initiating projects or activities due to a lack of self-confidence; going to extremes to seek nurturance and reassurance from others; feeling uncomfortable or helpless when left alone; and seeking to be in a relationship as soon as one ends in order to feel protected and supported. Though I do not discuss here the facet scores for this domain, it is notable to see how uniformly similar they are. This uniformity of high responses across the domain indicates that Agreeableness is a central and tightly organized dimension of Jennifer's personality.

Now we can look at her next highest score, a 57 (high) in Neuroticism. Neuroticism is concerned with emotional stability and, in particular, the tendency to experience negative affects, such as fear, sadness, anger, embarrassment, and guilt. Yet Neuroticism is also concerned with volatility in emotion, so it reflects individuals' tendencies to be impulsive, irrational, and to respond to stress poorly. Jennifer's high Neuroticism score indicates that she is more prone than the average female college student to periods of negative affect, which may result in bouts of impulsivity and vulnerability to stress. Notably, her Neuroti-

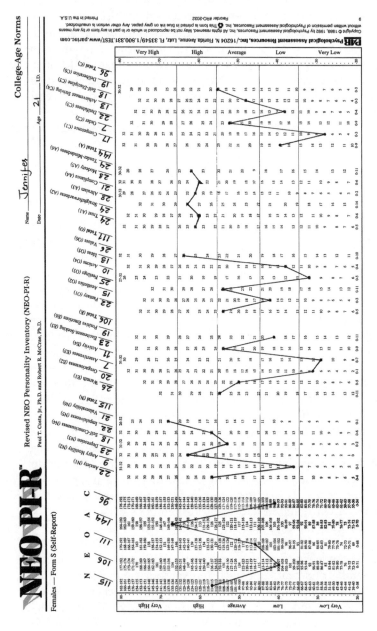

FIGURE 2.2. Jennifer's NEO PI-R profile. Profile form reproduced by special permission of the Publisher, Psychological Assessment Resources, Inc., 16204 North Florida Avenue, Lutz, Florida 33549, from the Revised NEO Personality Inventory by Paul T. Costa, Jr., PhD, and Robert R. McCrae, PhD. Copyright 1978, 1985, 1989, 1992 by PAR, Inc. Further reproduction is prohibited without permission from PAR, Inc.

cism profile shows a wide swing between her Vulnerability (very high) and her Angry Hostility (low). Overall high Neuroticism scores do not necessarily indicate a psychiatric disorder (especially when the respondents are being compared to a college-age nonclinical sample), but individuals with personality disorder features, ranging from obsessive-compulsive, histrionic, and dependent to narcissistic and borderline, are more likely to show elevated Neuroticism scores (Reynolds & Clark, 2001; Trull, 1992).

Turning to her low scores, Jennifer was below average on Extraversion (40—low) and Conscientiousness (41—low). The extraversion domain encompasses two related aspects—sociability and activity. Highly extraverted individuals tend to be energetic, optimistic, gregarious, and excitement-oriented. Individuals who score very low in this characteristic tend to be reserved, even-paced, and prefer to be alone. Extraverted individuals seek out situations that encourage positive emotion and lead to more pleasurable experiences. To score low in extraversion is to be prone to an absence of positive social encounters and opportunities in one's life. Yet once again, we must be careful in painting Jennifer's profile with too broad a brush. Her Extraversion score has three facets in the average range, one in the low range (Positive Emotion) and two in the very low range (Assertiveness and Activity). It would appear, then, that her Extraversion score divides up roughly along the sociability and active-assertiveness domains, with only the latter domain in the low area. We return to this critical difference shortly.

Her other low domain score is Conscientiousness, which encompasses the capacity for self-control, as demonstrated in "planning, organizing, and carrying out tasks" (Costa & McCrae, 1992, p. 16). It taps into individuals' achievement orientation, sense of competence, and diligence. Individuals who score high in this domain are likely to be successful in academics and occupations but may also tend toward compulsivity, fastidiousness, and overinvolvement in their work. Jennifer's low Conscientiousness score suggests that, at least in some areas of her life, she is experiencing herself as not in adequate control or effective in her activities. Once again, a closer analysis of the scatter in her facets for this domain will reveal additional information.

Finally, her Openness score falls in the average range. Openness is a dimension of curiosity and willingness to explore both one's internal world and the world of experience outside oneself. Open individuals enjoy new ideas, challenges, tastes, and cultural encounters. McCrae and Costa (1997) wrote that the quintessential high Openness individual is an artist or writer, yet they emphasize that Openness is only weakly to moderately correlated with standard measures of intelligence. The key qualities of Openness organize around a permeability of consciousness to experience and a desire to gain new experiences. In contrast, individuals who score very low in Openness would tend toward conventionality, narrowness in interests, and a preference for the familiar and the routine. Although Jennifer is low average in this domain, her facet scores reveal a wide scatter, with three facets that are low or very low (Aesthetics, Actions, and Ideas) and one facet, Values, that is high, bordering on very high. In fact, she is only in the average range for the two facets of Fantasy and Feelings. The overall scattered pattern in Openness provides helpful information for the emerging synthesis of Jennifer's scores and is further analyzed in the next section.

FACET ANALYSIS

Costa and McCrae (1992) encourage an analysis of the individual facets within each of the five dimensions, even though these facets all strongly correlate with the basic dimension to which they belong. They have found that the individual differences represented by these facets are stable and can be confirmed by observer ratings (McCrae & Costa, 1990, 2003). The facet analysis allows for more fine-grained understanding of the individual, including the opportunity to see patterns created by the facets across all the dimensions.

Agreeableness Facets

Jennifer's elevation on all six facets in this dimension makes its interpretation straightforward. In all aspects of sympathy and concern for others, depending on others, avoiding conflict, and self-effacement, Jennifer shows a pronounced preference and consistency.

Neuroticism Facets

Jennifer's most elevated facet in Neuroticism is Vulnerability. This means that she is prone to struggle under stress and is likely to feel dependent, hopeless, or panicky in these situations. Two other elevated facets, Anxiety and Depression, are fairly self-explanatory. Compared to other female college students, Jennifer is prone to worry, nervousness, and jittery feelings, as well as fears and phobias. She is also more likely to experience feelings of guilt, sadness, hopelessness, and loneliness. Her last elevated facet is Impulsivity, which refers to an inability to resist cravings or urges. Jennifer might be expected to give into desires for food, alcohol, cigarettes, possessions, but then to experience regret and guilt afterwards. Importantly, Jennifer also has one low facet in her otherwise high profile. Her low score in Angry Hostility indicates that she is slow to anger and unlikely to make hostile and negative attributions about others.

Extraversion Facets

Here, all of Jennifer's facets are in the average, low, and very low range. What is most striking, though, is the division in her scoring between those facets of Extraversion that emphasize interaction with others versus those that emphasize activity and energy. She is average in Gregariousness and even borders on high in Warmth, suggesting a genuine interest in and enjoyment of the company of others (which fits with her high Agreeableness scores). On the other hand, she is very low in Assertiveness, which implies deference to others and unwillingness to express her own desires. Similarly, she is low in Activity, which indicates unwillingness to move at a fast pace and take vigorous action. Finally, she is low in Positive Emotions, which points to a lowered capacity to seek out situations that bring her happiness, as well as a tendency to be less exuberant and high-spirited.

Conscientiousness Facets

Interestingly, the scatter of the facets reveals that Jennifer perceives herself in the average range in the aspects of Conscientiousness that refer to her intentions and thoughts. She sees herself as reasonably dutiful, self-disciplined, and capable of thinking ahead. However, in the three facets that express the results of these efforts in the external world (Competence, Order, and Achievement Striving), she experiences herself as low or very low. This difference may reflect a statement about her tendency to be self-critical and to judge her own efforts at competence in a rather harsh light.

Openness Facets

Here, we find some of the widest scatter in the profile, second only to the swings in Jennifer's Neuroticism profile. Her first three Openness facets fall in the average or just below average range. She shows average levels of imagination and proneness to fantasy, and creative daydreaming (Fantasy), as well as an average concern with and receptivity to her own feeling states and emotions (Feelings). She is just below average in her interest in and appreciation for art, music, and poetry (Aesthetics). Her very low score in Actions indicates that Jennifer finds change very challenging and much prefers to hold to her familiar routines and rituals. Her low score in Ideas points to Jennifer's limited interest in intellectual questions and lack of curiosity about unconventional or unorthodox ideas. On the other hand, her high score in Values suggests that Jennifer is not closed to political, social, or religious values that are different than her own. Given that she described herself as not being brought up in a strict religious background, this elevated score appears to be consistent with her self-presentation.

EXAMINING THE FACETS AND
DIMENSIONS IN COMBINATION

I have chosen Jennifer's profile in part because it yields a coherent and consistent picture of who she perceives herself to be as she stands on the brink of graduation from college. To pull this interpretation together, it is helpful to find the general patterns across all the facets. The NEO PI-R manual (Costa & McCrae, 1992) provides a factor analysis of all 30 facets for the five dimensions (Chapter 7, Table 5, p. 44), which allows one to see how facets cluster across the dimensions. In Jennifer's case, it is revealing to note that the Angry Hostility facet, which was her lowest score on the Neuroticism scale, loads powerfully in a negative direction on Agreeableness, her strongest dimension. In other words, Jennifer's lack of anger and her restraint in showing hostility to others are highly related to her tendency to be trusting of and compliant toward others. Similarly, Activity (which was her lowest score on Extraversion) loads positively on Conscientiousness, which was another low dimension for her. This link suggests that her lack of engagement in vigorous activity parallels her difficulties with feeling competent and successful in achievement striving. This point gets reinforced further when we see that Competence loads negatively on Neuroticism. Jennifer's low score on this facet of Conscientiousness only reinforces her high overall score on Neuroticism.

We next turn to an examination of pairings among the five dimensions, what Costa and McCrae (1992) call "personality styles" or "dimensional matrices" (see Costa & Piedmont, 2003, pp. 270–275; also see Piedmont, 1998, for research on these matrices). Originally, Costa and McCrae sought to locate the Big Five in relation to the well-researched work on underlying dimensions in interpersonal interactions (Leary, 1957; Wiggins, 1979, 2003; see also Chapter 5, this volume). This research had demonstrated that one could derive an "interpersonal circle" or "circumplex" that aligns individuals along two axes, one representing a continuum of Love (e.g., affiliation, trust, nurturance) and the other, Status (e.g., dominance, power, achievement). Any point on this circle represents the blend of these two qualities, with the relative weight of each dimension a function of the point's distance from the poles of each axis.

Costa and McCrae (1992) initially found that the interpersonal circle corresponds to the E and A dimensions of the NEO PI-R, with Extraversion capturing both high levels of Love and Status, while Agreeableness corresponds to a high Love and low Status orientation on the circle. Subsequently, they expanded this circumplex approach to find 10 different "personality styles" based on pairings of each of the Big Five dimensions (Costa & McCrae, 1998). For example, Figure 2.3 illustrates how what Costa and Piedmont (2003; Costa & McCrae, 1998) call "Styles of Interest" are made up of four quadrants that measure the joint contribution of Extraversion and Openness. Since Jennifer is low on Extraversion and on the low-average side of Openness, she would fall in the *Homebodies* quadrant, associating her with a preference for small groups and more unadventurous activities.

Paralleling this finding would be her Style of Interaction (E and A), which locates her in the E–A+ quadrant, *Unassuming*. This placement suggests that she is more likely to be modest and self-effacing, but also highly responsive to others' needs. At times, her trusting quality may lead others to take advantage of her.

The Style of Well-Being (N and E) pairs Jennifer's high N and low E (N+E–), and this is one of the most important findings for her, since it is associated with individuals who tend to be easily distressed and overwhelmed by pressure, as well as self-critical, insecure, and nervous (see Costa & McCrae, 1984; McCrae & Costa, 1991; Watson & Clark, 1997). Since many researchers (Barrett, 1997; McAdams, 2006; Watson & Tellegen, 1985) have equated Extraversion with the capacity to "feel good" in one's life, and Neuroticism with the opposing orientation to "feel bad," Jennifer is likely to allow negative affects to overwhelm the positive experiences in her life. The quadrant's designation of *Gloomy Pessimist* seems particularly apt.

Turning to her Style of Defense (N and O), Jennifer, with her N+ and low-average O, falls just within the *Maladaptive* (N+O–) quadrant, where individuals are more inclined to use denial and avoidance with regard to their negative feelings, as opposed to talking them out or exploring insights or solutions that will allow them to change and feel better.

Her Style of Anger Control (N and A) places her solidly in the *Timid* quadrant. Individuals within this grouping are conflicted over their anger. They may be easily hurt but are reluctant to express their frustration or identify the targets of their irritation. Unfortunately, it is not uncommon to redirect the anger inward.

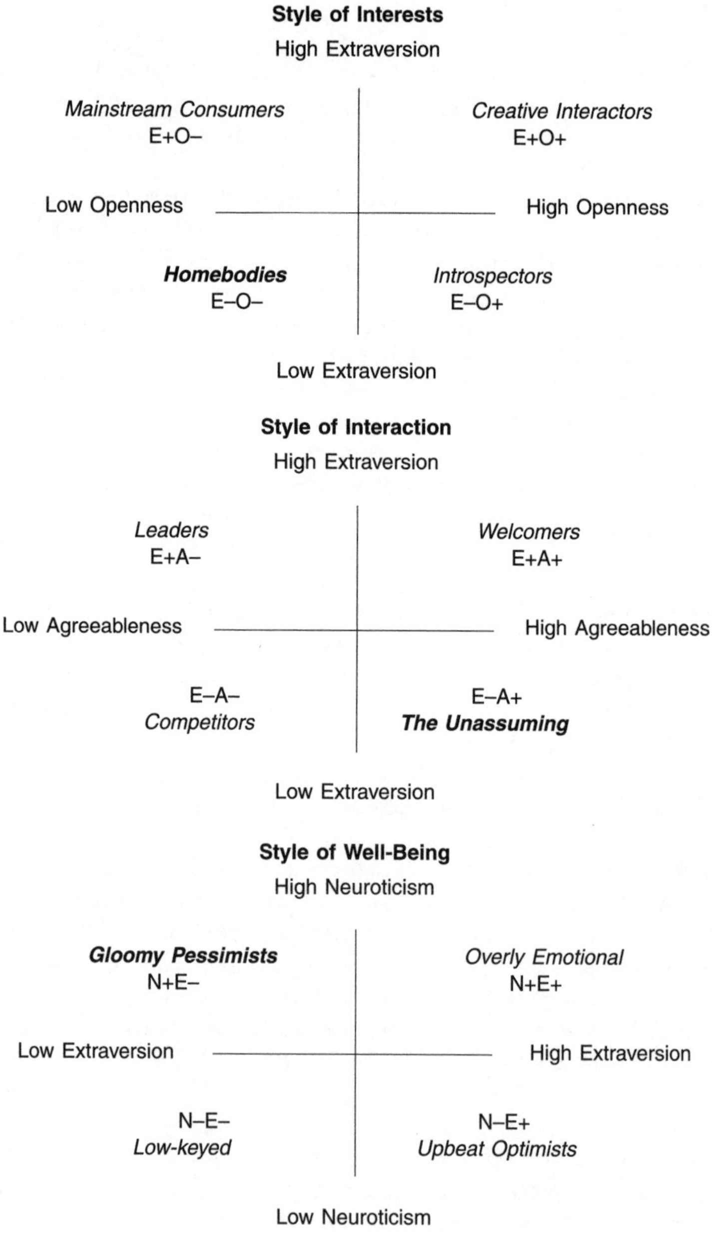

Style of Interests

High Extraversion

Mainstream Consumers
E+O–

Creative Interactors
E+O+

Low Openness ———————————— High Openness

Homebodies
E–O–

Introspectors
E–O+

Low Extraversion

Style of Interaction

High Extraversion

Leaders
E+A–

Welcomers
E+A+

Low Agreeableness ———————————— High Agreeableness

E–A–
Competitors

E–A+
The Unassuming

Low Extraversion

Style of Well-Being

High Neuroticism

Gloomy Pessimists
N+E–

Overly Emotional
N+E+

Low Extraversion ———————————— High Extraversion

N–E–
Low-keyed

N–E+
Upbeat Optimists

Low Neuroticism

FIGURE 2.3. Jennifer's personality styles from the NEO PI-R. Style graphs adapted by special permission of the Publisher, Psychological Assessment Resources, Inc., 16204 North Florida Avenue, Lutz, Florida 33549, from the Revised NEO Personality Inventory by Paul T. Costa, Jr., PhD, and Robert R. McCrae, PhD. Copyright 1978, 1985, 1989, 1992 by PAR, Inc. Further reproduction is prohibited without permission from PAR, Inc.

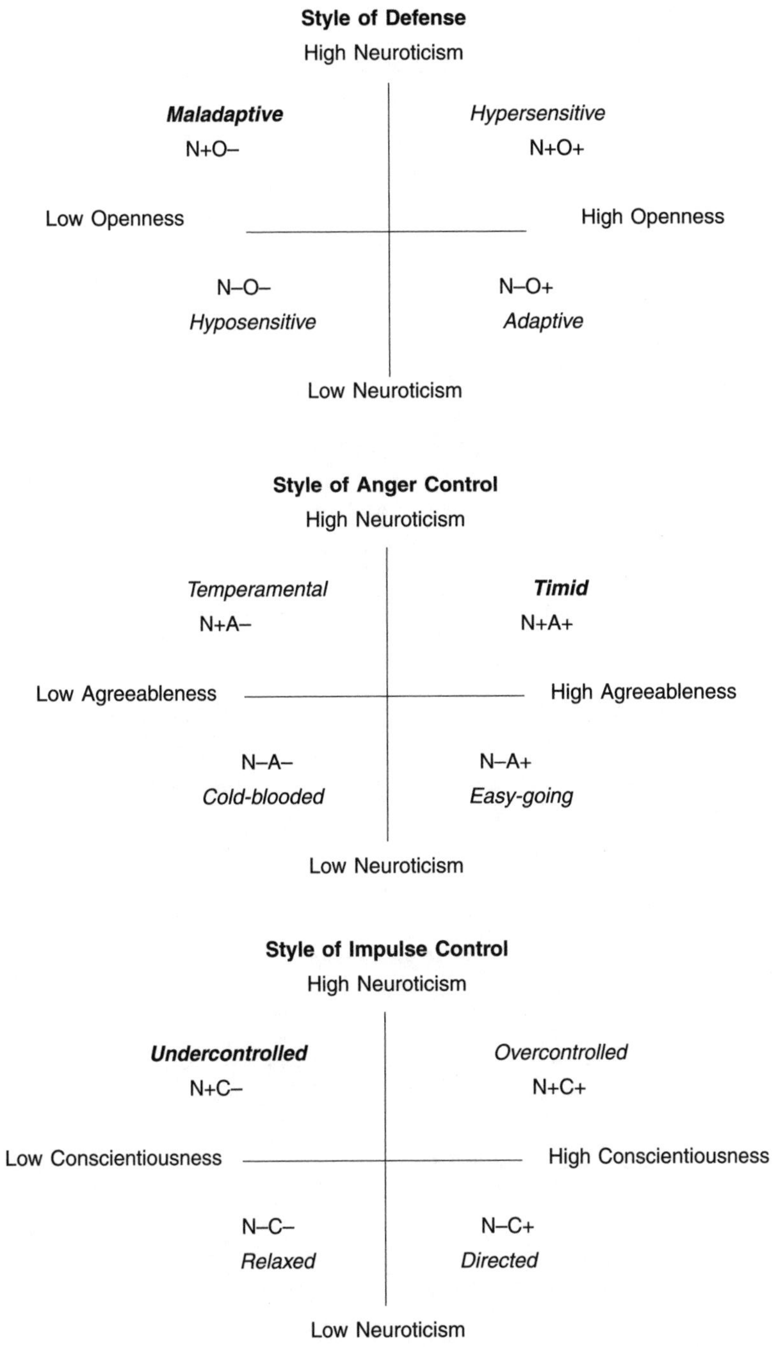

Style of Defense

High Neuroticism

Maladaptive
N+O–

Hypersensitive
N+O+

Low Openness ———————————— High Openness

N–O–
Hyposensitive

N–O+
Adaptive

Low Neuroticism

Style of Anger Control

High Neuroticism

Temperamental
N+A–

Timid
N+A+

Low Agreeableness ———————— High Agreeableness

N–A–
Cold-blooded

N–A+
Easy-going

Low Neuroticism

Style of Impulse Control

High Neuroticism

Undercontrolled
N+C–

Overcontrolled
N+C+

Low Conscientiousness ———————— High Conscientiousness

N–C–
Relaxed

N–C+
Directed

Low Neuroticism

FIGURE 2.3. *(continued)*

39

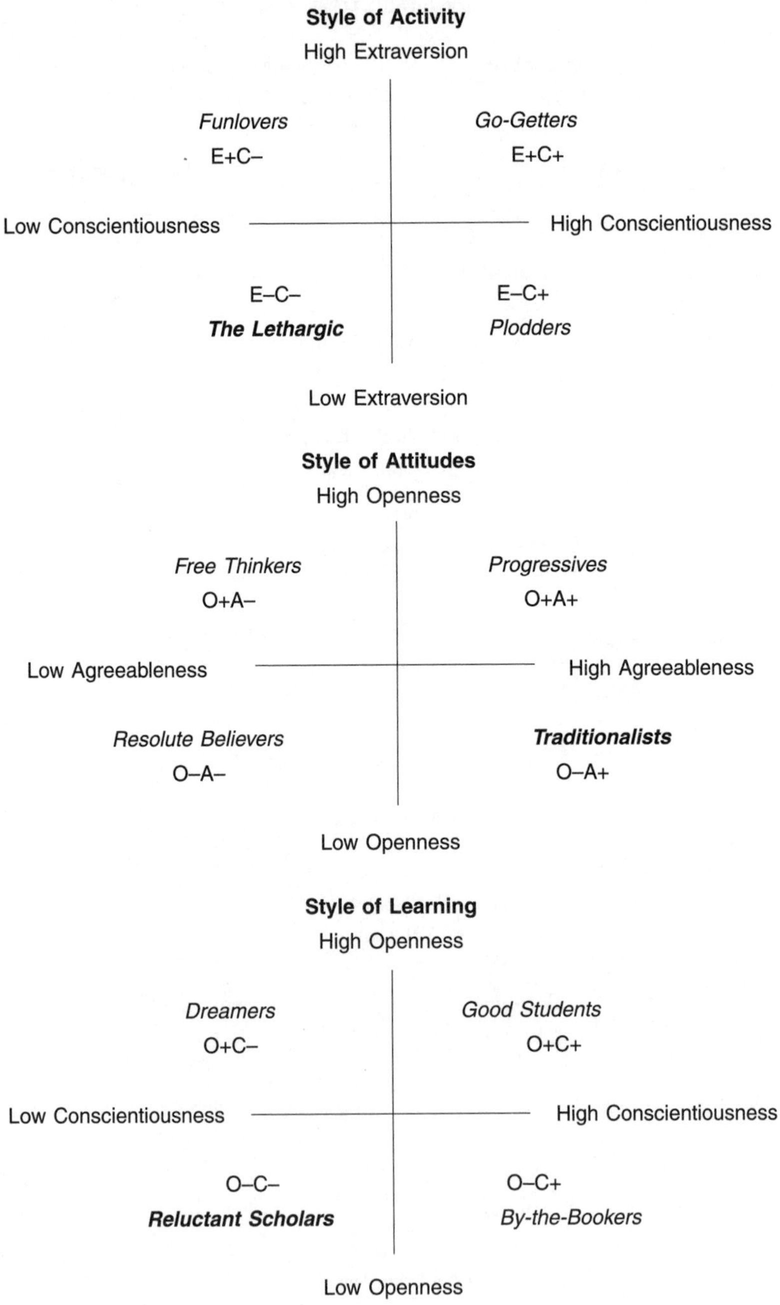

Style of Activity

High Extraversion

Funlovers	*Go-Getters*
E+C−	E+C+

Low Conscientiousness ———————————— High Conscientiousness

E−C−	E−C+
The Lethargic	*Plodders*

Low Extraversion

Style of Attitudes

High Openness

Free Thinkers	*Progressives*
O+A−	O+A+

Low Agreeableness ———————————— High Agreeableness

Resolute Believers	**Traditionalists**
O−A−	O−A+

Low Openness

Style of Learning

High Openness

Dreamers	*Good Students*
O+C−	O+C+

Low Conscientiousness ———————————— High Conscientiousness

O−C−	O−C+
Reluctant Scholars	*By-the-Bookers*

Low Openness

FIGURE 2.3. (*continued*)

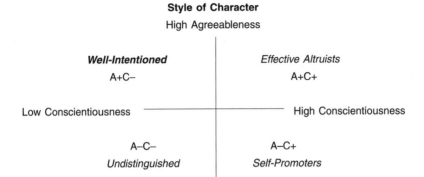

Style of Character

High Agreeableness

Well-Intentioned   *Effective Altruists*
A+C–   A+C+

Low Conscientiousness ——————————|—————————— High Conscientiousness

A–C–   A–C+
Undistinguished   *Self-Promoters*

Low Agreeableness

FIGURE 2.3. (*continued*)

Her Impulse Control Style (N and C) identifies her in the *Undercontrolled* Category (N+C–). Due to her lowered sense of self-control and anxiety, Jennifer is particularly prone to give in to momentary impulses and is likely to engage in substance abuse and other risky health behaviors.

Jennifer's Style of Activity (E and C) score places her in the *Lethargic* (E–C–) category, which, again, may be a reflection of depressed mood state. Individuals in this grouping have few plans or goals to motivate them. They tend toward passivity and only rally to the most imminent demands. They tend to lag behind in and avoid group-based activities.

With her low-average O and high A score Jennifer's Style of Attitudes (O and A) edges into the *Traditionalist* quadrant, which associates her with individuals who rely on the values of their family and tend to like established rules and routines as the best approach to life.

Her Styles of Learning (O and C) pairing lands her just within the designation of the *Reluctant Scholar* quadrant (O–C–). These individuals are not naturally inclined to intellectual or academic pursuits. They may require extra assistance to stay on task and meet the demands of their assigned work. Their interests tend to veer in directions other than scholarly endeavors.

Last, Jennifer's Style of Character (A and C) locates her firmly in the *Well-Intentioned* quadrant (A+C–). She is among individuals who tend to be accepting and see the best in others, but who can be easily swayed in their judgments and not always consistent in their decisions. They are giving and concerned about others but do not always follow through on good intentions, and they end up relying more on the kindness of others.

Pulling all of this information together, I can make a formulation of Jennifer's personality at this first domain of Basic Tendencies. To do so, I can consider the fundamental aspects of personality—cognition, affect, motivation, and behavior.

OVERALL PERSONALITY INTERPRETATION

Beginning with her affective or emotional style, Jennifer shows a strong tendency toward depressive and anxious feelings, as well as an extreme vulnerability to being overwhelmed by stress and pressure. Her emotional state may result in behavioral difficulties with asserting herself, taking action, and successfully placing herself in situations that will lift her mood and bring positive emotion into her life. Her negative emotions and inability to regulate them may contribute to cognitions of self-criticism and diminished self-confidence. This discomfort with herself may contribute to her self-perception that she is disorganized, does not follow through on plans and decisions, and has not achieved the level of competency in school, athletics, or work that she desires. In response to these uncomfortable feelings and self-perceptions, she may give into momentary impulses that provide short-term pleasure but end up causing her to feel regret and additional self-condemnation. This cycle of negative affects, cognitions, and behaviors may undermine Jennifer's sense of autonomy, motivating her to seek out others for support and guidance. Paradoxically, this dependence on others comes at a time when the demand for her to demonstrate independence and maturity, given her incipient graduation from college, is greatest. On the positive side, her warmth and ability to trust in others make Jennifer likely to make successful connections with others and to maintain positive relationships.

Given her comfort with tried and tested routines, and her lack of openness to new experiences and ideas, Jennifer may be at a disadvantage for extricating herself from the negative cycle that she has entered. On the one hand, combined with her lack of assertiveness and tendency to be dependent, this preference for familiarity may lead her to stay too long in relationships or to continue to lean on her parents, brother, and hometown friends. A certain level of rigidity may block her opportunity for self-generated creative solutions to her current stressors and depressed feelings. On the other hand, as long as Jennifer can structure a safe and unthreatening world, nurtured by intimate family and friends, she is likely to minimize stress, function competently, and enjoy warm and supportive relationships. Unfortunately, societal pressure in our culture at this phase of Jennifer's life demands that she articulate plans for an independent future, "leave the nest," and forge a professional or occupational identity. Her profile does not provide evidence that she is making much headway on this path. Her awareness of this fact may contribute to her depressed and anxious state.

WHAT IS MISSING?

Whenever I dive into a personality analysis based on the NEO PI-R, I am stunned by the depth and complexity of information that a 30- to 40-minute questionnaire can provide. It is a great credit to Costa and McCrae's (1992; McCrae & Costa, 2003) thoughtful synthesis of many decades of personality study and psychometric work. With the burgeoning validation literature on the Big Five (McCrae & Costa, 1987; McCrae & John, 1992), I can also feel assured that the profile of Jennifer is not only reliable but also likely to be successful in predicting her responses across a variety of situations. We have learned about a number of the affective, cognitive, and behavioral factors that are not only most prominent for Jennifer as she prepares to finish her college years but also suggestive of the contours of her adult life. Longitudinal studies of the Big Five tend to find stability in these traits over the life course, though Neuroticism scores in general decline, while the traits related to social and vocational competence (Agreeableness and Conscientiousness, respectively) show higher scores from early adulthood to midlife (Aldwin & Levensen, 1994; McCrae et al., 2000). Still, while Jennifer is likely to continue to develop and change, her responses to the NEO PI-R may indeed reflect a core foundation of her basic cognitive–affective and behavioral tendencies.

Within the trait assessment approach I have used, one factor that is missing in order to achieve a comprehensive assessment is an observer's ratings on Form R of the NEO PI-R. For example, it would be extremely informative to know how a roommate, boyfriend, parent, or sibling might have rated Jennifer on the five dimensions. Even though observer ratings for the most part agree with self-reports (Costa & Piedmont, 2003) and discrepancies are more often due to different interpretations of words and items than to large variances in judgments (McCrae, Stone, Fagan, & Costa, 1998), there is still a unique vantage point provided by someone outside the respondent's perceptions. An observer's ratings provide a valuable window into the public persona of the respondent and how others may receive his or her intended behaviors in unintended ways. Still, Costa and Piedmont (2003, p. 265) stress that the observer's ratings should not be considered the "gold standard" for judging the personality of the respondent when discrepancies arise. The respondent has access to many more situations for self-observation than even the most intimate observer, not to mention access to internal states; therefore, the observer's viewpoint suffers its own limitations with respect to the respondent's views. McCrae (1993) suggests that when the examiner receives discrepant results, it is best to go back to the respondent and the observer and to use these differences as forum for discussion and more nuanced understanding of the individual. In Chapter 7, I illustrate this approach in my work with a husband and wife in couple therapy. Once again, since neither partner has a corner on the truth in either self- or other-perceptions, the nature of the discrepancies between viewpoints says much about the communication and synchrony of the relationship. On the other hand, in situations in which one cannot return to the respondent and the observer to explore reasons for discrepancies, McCrae recommends that the best course is to average the ratings and use the merged profile for interpretation. In summary, if one goes ahead and uses the NEO PI-R in practice, obtaining both type of ratings is optimal, but there is still much that can be learned (as we have seen) from receiving only the self-ratings.

But leaving these trait assessment considerations aside, what else is missing? Is this the whole of Jennifer? In pondering this question, consider the way that McCrae and Costa (2003) ended the second edition of their influential book *Personality in Adulthood: A Five-Factor Theory Perspective*. To discuss the application of the five-factor perspective to an understanding of an individual's life narrative and identity, they selected the autobiography, *The Confessions*, by the great political theorist and writer, Jean-Jacques Rousseau (1781/1953). Building on the ratings of Rousseau by political scientist and biographer A. M. Melzer (cited in McCrae, 1996), they applied a five-factor interpretation both to Rousseau's behavior and to the content and quality of his autobiography. For example, they found that Rousseau was extremely high in Neuroticism and Openness, while low in Agreeableness and Conscientiousness, and then postulated,

> Is it surprising that one so high in Openness to Feelings would be one of the founders of the Romantic Movement in literature or that one so low in Trust but so high in Tender-mindedness would reject the political philosophy of the day and offer his own Utopian alternative in *The Social Contract* . . . ? (McCrae & Costa, 2003, p. 233)

I do not mean to be too ironic in quoting this passage, but, clearly, knowing Rousseau's five-factor profile does not make his generation of a lasting work of genius any less surprising. It is fair to say that over the nearly 230 years since he lived and the billions of people who have lived and died, there have been numerous individuals who might have received NEO PI-R profiles that would have approximated the same pattern of ratings Melzer applied to Rousseau. Yet we can be equally sure that not one of those individuals was likely to author *The Social Contract, The Confessions,* or *Émile.* In a sense, it might be *necessary* to imagine that Rousseau would display this type of profile to generate the groundbreaking and convention-smashing work that he did, but his profile is hardly *sufficient* to explain the course of his life and writings. To understand the production of his masterpieces, we would need to know much more about how this work grew out of his life experiences, the particular political pressures of his era, and his own goals and aspirations in his life. McCrae and Costa (2003) themselves clearly acknowledge the need for an understanding of these structures (their five-factor theory includes Characteristic Adaptations and the Self-Concept, along with demographic and biographical influences), and it is to these types of higher order structures of the personality that we must turn.

To know that Jennifer is high in Agreeableness and Neuroticism and low in Extraversion and Conscientiousness may set some limits on what we might expect or predict about her behavior, but how are each of these aspects expressed in the actual life that she has lived and will live? How are they manifested in the *roles, situations, time periods,* and *developmental phases* that constitute the lived experience of her life (McAdams, 2006, p. 8)? In summary, we may know about the frame of Jennifer's personality, but not what fills out its picture, color, and texture.

From what we know so far, Jennifer could be extremely dependent on a boyfriend, roommate, parent, her brother, or some combination of all of these individuals. Does she express her dependency in one or all of the *roles* of girlfriend, friend, daughter, or sister? Does her diminished sense of competence manifest itself in all the roles she adopts in life and in all areas?

In what *situations* does Jennifer express her vulnerability to stress? Is she prone to avoid competition in her academic work but not on the playing field? Does she thrive in her friendships but find the social world of dating and parties difficult to handle? In what situations does she display her impulsivity, and how? Does she let go impulsively in parties, shopping malls, dining halls, casinos, or speeding in a car?

Additionally, we do not know Jennifer's unique *goals* or aspirations. We do not know what she *wants* and is *typically trying to do* in her life. For example, when Jennifer judges herself as not competent or striving for achievement, is this a realistic appraisal, or is it the appraisal of an individual who sets high standards and judges herself harshly when she does not live up to them? Is her warmth and sympathy toward others a genuine expression of her compassion and tender heartedness, or is it a reflection of need and insecurity? By knowing Jennifer's stated goals, we have a better understanding of her low score in Conscientiousness and her elevated score in Agreeableness. This knowledge might indeed provide insight into her elevated Neuroticism score.

We also need to know more about how Jennifer employs *defenses* in her life to protect against her vulnerability to stress and her proneness to anxiety and depression. We have some information that she may narrow her life to zones of comfort and reach out to others for help in coping, and that she may be inclined toward avoidance or denial, but we have little sense about the breadth of these defenses and in what specific situations she will be likely to apply them. The NEO PI-R offers us a wide sampling of thoughts, behaviors, and potential defenses, but it makes no causal links to explain how these different aspects of Jennifer might be connected and in what situations or times they might be applied.

Finally, I have emphasized that the portrayal of Jennifer we have fashioned catches her at a time of transition in her life. Even if her profile were to remain consistent at various junctures in her life, in what ways might it be subtly affected by the particular *time period* and *developmental phases* of her life? A few years later, perhaps comfortably immersed in a new community and working in a rewarding job, would Jennifer provide a profile that would reflect an enhanced sense of her competence and a reduced expression of negative emotion? To gain greater insight into the questions, we would want to know more about Jennifer's own developmental history and background. Were there indeed periods in which she had different perceptions of herself, a different balance of positive and negative emotion, or a different approach to her social relationships?

Returning to the fundamental aspects of McAdams's Domain 2, we need to know about Jennifer's goals and defenses in the context of the diverse roles, situations, and time periods that constitute the textured contexts of her life. To approach knowledge of Jennifer's whole person, we need to turn to an analysis of the where, when, and how of her personality, not simply the "what" that the NEO PI-R provides. To answer these questions more effectively, I turn to measures that belong in the second domain of Characteristic Adaptations. In this way, we begin to fill out our picture of Jennifer in the context of her unique life aspirations and the settings that form the backdrop for these wishes, dreams, and fears.

3

Domain 2—
Characteristic Adaptations

Personal Strivings and Defenses

In the acclaimed novel *Cold Mountain* (Frazier, 1997/2003), made into the highly successful film starring Nicole Kidman and Jude Law, we follow the desperate efforts of the protagonist Inman to make his way back from a Civil War hospital to his home in a mountain community of North Carolina. Though the demands of realism forced the film to give Inman a first name and to embody him with an actor's physical presence, the novel stubbornly kept the details of his identity and his physical characteristics to an absolute minimum. Inman personifies "everyman," and his journey expresses the universal longings for home and romantic love that live *in man* and are heightened by deprivations of war. To the extent that we come to know about Inman's character, it is only through the desires he expresses, the goals he sets, and the actions that he takes. Inman is a man striving toward a clear purpose—to reunite with Ada in Cold Mountain. In the end, however, our knowledge of this simple purpose is sufficient to make us care intensely about him and the outcome of his quest, despite the fact that we cannot name the color of his eyes or describe the sound of his voice.

In contrast, a 19th-century novelist such as Charles Dickens is more likely to build a character from the description of observable mannerisms and physical characteristics. For example, here is how we first meet

Uriah Heep, the infamous, unctuous villain from *David Copperfield*, who engages in a series of sinister manipulations throughout the novel:

> The low arched door then opened, and the face came out. It was quite cadaverous as it had looked in the window. . . . It belonged to a red-haired person—a youth of fifteen, as I take it now, but looking much older—whose hair was cropped as close as the closest stubble, who had hardly any eyebrows, and no eyelashes, and eyes of red-brown, so unsheltered and unshaded, that I remember wondering how he went to sleep. He was high-shouldered and bony, dressed in decent black, with a white wisp of a neckcloth, buttoned up to the throat, and had a long lank skeleton hand, which particularly attracted my attention, as he stood . . . rubbing his chin with it, and looking up at us. . . . (Dickens, 1869/1962, pp. 224–225)

From this description, we can immediately infer the saturnine nature that fundamentally characterizes Heep, despite his superficial efforts to express humility and courtesy. He literally appears to be rising from the "low-arched" door of a crypt and poking his "cadaverous" head toward David.

These two equally effective and markedly different approaches to conveying central characters in works of fiction place in clear relief the fundamental difference between the first and second domains of McAdams's framework of personality research. In the previous chapter, I sought to describe Jennifer in terms of her stable traits of temperament, interpersonal style, and self-discipline. I painted a picture of *who* she is in the same way that Dickens builds an initial characterization of Uriah Heep. Now, in this chapter, I turn to a depiction of Jennifer that is based not so much in description of her attributes, but rather in an exploration of her desires and efforts to obtain her strivings. We look not so much at what she is like, but at what she is *trying to do*. In addition to examining her strivings, we also study how she protects herself from the frustration of these goals and how she seeks to avoid her most feared outcomes.

This balancing act between seeking to fulfill one's most urgent goals and the accommodative strategies one employs in light of frustration has been dubbed *self-regulation* (Brown, 1998; Carver & Scheier, 1981, 1998; Higgins, 1987, 1997, 1998) and is indeed one of the central paradigms of contemporary personality research. In any self-regulatory model of personality, it is hypothesized that individuals set a standard that directs or guides behavior toward its ideal (Carver & Scheier, 1998, 1999). Individuals rely on a "comparator" system to evaluate their current status in light of the standard they have set. Depending on the degree and rate of progress, individuals generate emotional and behavioral responses that feed back into the system, creating further reductions or increases in the discrepancies from the standard. According to this model of personality, to understand people, we must know more about the particular goals they have set for themselves in their lives and then ascertain the progress they perceive they are making toward the fulfillment of these goals. This is exactly the task I have set to accomplish in the next steps in finding out about the personality of Jennifer.

To uncover the force of goals in Jennifer's current life, we could explore her most fundamental motives of achievement, power, affiliation, and intimacy, as measured through analysis of Thematic Apperception Test (TAT) stories (Atkinson, Heyns, & Veroff, 1954; Boyatzis, 1973; McAdams, 1984; McClelland, 1961; Murray, 1938; Smith, 1992; Winter, 1973; Woike, Gershkovich, Piorkowski, & Polo, 1999). Knowing Jennifer's degree of achievement motive or her affiliation motive would certainly take us a step beyond the "what she is" aspects of her personality that we have tapped through our trait analysis. We would fill in the deeper picture of *why* she tends to be so trusting or agreeable, as opposed to identifying her simply in these descriptive terms. Yet such basic motives are still intended to be broad personality constructs from which one can derive a series of more specific and contextualized motivational constructs (Emmons, 1989). Additionally, scoring of these motives through the TAT requires a reasonable degree of training, which is appropriate for research projects but may be too time-consuming for general clinicians who want a more accessible and streamlined approach to evaluating the motivational concerns of their patients. There also continues to be controversy over the clinical utility of the TAT for both diagnosis and prediction (Lilienfeld, Wood, & Garb, 2000; but see also Karon, 2000).

For our purposes, then, it would be attractive to find a way to measure Jennifer's motivation in a more concrete and direct fashion. Robert Emmons (1986, 1989, 1999) has introduced the concept of "personal strivings" for exactly this purpose. In characterizing the motivational system, he described it as being the system of the personality that is concerned with what individuals are trying to accomplish in their lives— what they seek to gain, and what they seek to avoid. He proposed that personal strivings exist at a middle level in a hierarchical model of motivation (see Figure 3.1). At the highest level of motivation are the fundamental motives I have just mentioned. At the next level are personal strivings that define motives in more specific categories of action, yet remain relatively abstract and flexible ("strive for fame and fortune," "raise a loving family," "live a moral life"). The third level consists of more time-bound and context-based goals—Klinger's (1999) current concerns, Little's personal projects (1989, 1999), and Cantor's develop-

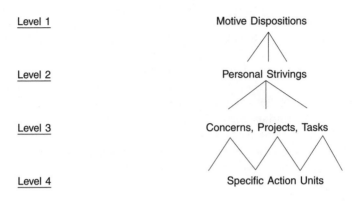

Level 1   Motive Dispositions

Level 2   Personal Strivings

Level 3   Concerns, Projects, Tasks

Level 4   Specific Action Units

FIGURE 3.1. Hierarchical model of motivation. From *The Remembered Self: Emotion and Memory in Personality* by Jefferson A. Singer and Peter Salovey (p. 61, 72). Copyright 1993 by Jefferson A. Singer and Peter Salovey. Reprinted with permission of The Free Press, a Division of Simon & Schuster Adult Publishing Group. All rights reserved.

mental life tasks (Cantor, Norem, Niedenthal, Langston, & Brower, 1987). The fourth level defines specific behaviors and sequences of actions in which individuals engage to achieve the fulfillment of their projects and tasks (Schank & Abelson, 1977).

As Emmons (1989) indicated, all of these models share Murray's (1938) original notion of *subsidiation* (what he called *actones*, or specific actions growing from needs that are in turn driven by complexes), which means the instrumental relationship of one motive construct leading to the next and the next at increasing levels of specificity and concreteness. For a similar perspective, one can look at Carver and Scheier's concept of goal hierarchies (1998) or Vallacher and Wegner's (1987) *action identification theory.*

For example (following Figure 3.1), an individual high in an intimacy motive (Level 1) holds the personal striving of seeking a romantic partner (Level 2). This striving leads to frequent thoughts of dating and romance, which culminate in a personal project of finding a girlfriend when he leaves for college (Level 3). The confluence of his developmental life task and his interest in a personal project directs his specific actions (Level 4) toward attending a variety of first-year mixers, joining several college activities, and spending long hours cultivating his personal appearance. In this sense, each motive–action at the next level of the hierarchy takes its cue from the one above it in the sequence. In other words, the motivational system is best characterized by its capacity to organize the biological, cognitive, and affective systems into coordinated sequences of instrumental actions in pursuit of a specific goal, activated internally or externally.

According to this view of the hierarchy of motivational constructs, personal strivings offer an ideal "middle level" construct (Emmons, 1989) to measure Jennifer's goal orientations. If we look at her specific scripted actions (Schank & Abelson, 1977), we might know a great deal about Jennifer's most immediate preoccupations and activities, but we might not grasp the larger picture of her enduring personality that we are seeking. If we studied her engagement with particular personal projects or life tasks (in this case, graduating college and embarking on living independently), we certainly could study her unique responses to these challenges, but our analysis would be driven more by the context of these events than by Jennifer's long-standing characteristics. And, as I have already suggested, an analysis of her fundamental motives at the highest level of the hierarchy would leave us at a similar decontextualized level of abstraction that is too similar to our Domain 1— Trait Perspective. Examining individuals' personal strivings by looking at what they "typically try to do" allows us to get at both their long-standing motivational concerns and behavioral tendencies that are likely to be tied to particular situations, roles, and time periods that provide the additional level of context that we seek. So with regard to our goal of building up a picture of Jennifer that is reasonably comprehensive, stable, and context-specific, they offer an especially effective and practical tool for our work.

COLLECTING PERSONAL STRIVINGS

To explore Jennifer's personal strivings, we used the Emmons personal striving assessment method (Emmons, 1986) and asked Jennifer to consider "the things that you typically or characteristically are trying to do in everyday behavior." We provided her with examples, such as "trying to persuade others one is right" or "trying to help others in need of help" (Emmons, 1997). We told her that she should not focus on how successful she might be in a particular striving, but simply on how typically and frequently she pursued it. We also explained that the strivings should not be one-time concerns, but should be goal activities in which she engages on a regular basis. As is typical in personal striving research, we presented her with a sheet that contained 15 stems beginning with "I typically try to. . . ."

After Jennifer finished writing down her strivings, we provided her with a Striving Assessment Matrix. This consisted of a set of ratings that Jennifer made for each striving. In Emmons's (1986) original striving assessment work, participants filled out 16 different rating scales for each striving that they had listed. Emmons (1997) has indicated that across the motivational literature, ratings of goals or strivings usually yield a few basic dimensions that represent the underlying organization of how individuals think about their goals. Factor analyses from several studies (e.g., Cantor & Langston, 1989; Emmons, 1986; Ruehlman & Wolchik, 1988) have converged on three robust dimensions (Emmons, 1997, p. 500):

1. The degree of commitment/investment in the goal.
2. The degree to which the goal is perceived as stressful/challenging.
3. The anticipated outcome/reward.

Emmons (1989, 1997) has referred to these dimensions as Commitment/Intensity, Ease/Effort, and Desirability/Reward. Commitment/Intensity encompasses the importance of the goal—its value and significance to the individual. Ease/Effort captures the difficulty that the individual anticipates experiencing in pursuit of the goal, as well as an estimate of the probability of its attainment. Desirability/Reward includes the affective dimension of the goal—how happy one would be to achieve it, how sad if one failed in its attainment, or how many ambivalent or conflicted feelings one has regarding its pursuit.

In working with the students from my seminar, I asked them to look over the 16 rating scales that Emmons used and to select a subset that would fit their participant best, based on the NEO PI-R results. However, I also asked that they make sure that the subset they selected covered the three fundamental dimensions that Emmons had identified. In the case of Jennifer, we ended up using the following six Striving Assessment Dimensions—Happiness on Striving Attainment; Unhappiness on Striving Nonattainment; Ambivalence about Striving Attainment; Commitment to the Striving; Success in Past Month of Attainment; and Probability of Successful Attainment in the Future. The first three dimensions tapped into Desirability, the fourth, into Commitment, and the final two, into Ease/Effort. These six dimensions in the columns and the 13 strivings in the row form a Striving Assessment Matrix, as depicted in Table 3.3 (p. 61; rating scales for each dimension and the wording and anchors associated with each scale are listed). Jennifer was asked to fill out all six ratings for each of the strivings she recorded, forming a potential matrix of 90 ratings (though she made only 78 ratings due to generating 13 instead of 15 strivings).

Before I review this analysis of Jennifer's strivings and ratings, let me point out that clinicians can gain much from simply asking for 10 personal strivings, then having the client do three simple ratings for Commitment (Importance), Reward (Happiness), and Difficulty (Ease/ Effort). Once clients have recorded their 10 strivings, they then can rate each one on a 0- to 6-point scale for how *important* it is to them, how much *happiness* it would bring on attainment, and how *difficult* it would be to attain. As we shall see with Jennifer, examinations of patterns across these three dimensions can reveal relationships among the importance placed on a striving, the imagined happiness that its attainment would bring, and the relative possibility of actually making the striving a reality. In my Chapter 7 case presentation in this volume, I provide a straightforward demonstration of an application of this type of personal striving assessment in clinical practice. For now, in the spirit of our more comprehensive understanding of Jennifer, we engage in a more extensive analysis of her strivings.

SCORING THE CONTENT OF PERSONAL STRIVINGS

Approach and Avoidance

Table 3.1 displays the strivings that Jennifer wrote down. She asked to stop at 13, indicating that she would be straining to list an additional two. One basic way to look at her striving content is to examine how many of the strivings are approach-oriented and how many are avoidance-

TABLE 3.1. Jennifer's Personal Strivings

1. I typically try to . . . avoid situations that make me uncomfortable.
2. I typically try to . . . make others feel comfortable.
3. I typically try to . . . spend as much as time with my family as possible.
4. I typically try to . . . find ways to improve my self-esteem.
5. I typically try to . . . do work in advance in order to avoid stress.
6. I typically try to . . . make other people feel good about themselves.
7. I typically try to . . . be open-minded about others' views.
8. I typically try to . . . avoid people who view me negatively.
9. I typically try to . . . improve my appearance.
10. I typically try to . . . remain in a familiar environment (or one that makes me comfortable).
11. I typically try to . . . be on time to my engagements.
12. I typically try to . . . avoid feeling inferior in terms of intelligence (seeming unintelligent).
13. I typically try to . . . avoid judging others.

based. Research has demonstrated that individuals who are inclined to value avoidance goals are more prone to Neuroticism and to have memories related to phobic concerns (Elliot, Sheldon, & Church, 1997; Moffitt & Singer, 1994; Singer, 1990). In previous research (Moffitt & Singer, 1994), I found that most participants provide no more than one or two avoidance strivings out of a set of 15. Jennifer listed 5 out of 13 (strivings 1, 5, 8, 12, and 13) and at least one other (10) that could be considered to be as much about avoiding discomfort as about striving for something positive. If we include striving 10 as an avoidance goal, this total amounts to 46% of her strivings, which places her toward the extreme of individuals for avoidance goals.

Next let us consider the nature of what Jennifer seeks to avoid. She wants to avoid situations that make her uncomfortable, academic stress, people who view her negatively, feeling or seeming unintelligent, and judging others. Taking this last striving in tandem with her striving to be "open-minded about others' views," we see confirmation of her high Values facet score on the Openness dimension of the NEO PI-R. She is truly invested in not judging others harshly or dismissing their points of view simply because they may differ from her own. Given her concern about how her appearance and intelligence are perceived by others, it may be that Jennifer hopes in return that others will withhold from critical or narrow-minded judgments of her.

Jennifer's other avoidance goals also correspond to facet scores that she received on the NEO PI-R. Her elevated anxiety and vulnerability to stress scores on the Neuroticism scale fit closely with her strivings to avoid uncomfortable situations and critical individuals, as well her desire to minimize academic pressure. Her striving to avoid appearing unintelligent aligns with her doubts about her own competence and achievement striving, as measured by the Conscientiousness dimension.

In turning to Jennifer's approach strivings, it is striking how they also link to her NEO PI-R high scores on Agreeableness and Neuroticism and lower scores on Extraversion and Openness. Jennifer seeks "to make others feel comfortable," "make other people feel good about themselves," and "be on time to engagements." At the same time, she wants "to spend as much time with her family as possible" (while also remaining in familiar environments that make her comfortable). We see here not only her uniform Agreeableness expressed in her accommodation, trustworthiness, and kindness to others, which indicates warmth toward other people, but also a desire to avoid conflict or impose on others. Her interest in her family and living a life high in "familiarity" reflects her lack of Assertiveness, as well as her low facet scores on Openness for Actions and Ideas.

Her other two approach strivings—"find ways to improve my self-esteem" and "improve my appearance"—are also consistent with her NEO PI-R profile. The goals of improving self-esteem and appearance, by definition, indicate her evaluation that each condition is not adequate and must be enhanced. This dissatisfaction with herself—both externally and internally—is a cornerstone of elevated depression and a lowered sense of personal competence, both of which Jennifer displayed on her NEO PI-R facet scores.

Motivational Themes

Another way to evaluate the strivings' content is to code them for their motivational themes. Emmons (1989, 1999) has developed a coding manual for identifying 12 overarching motivational themes across individuals' sets of strivings. Each theme conveys a distinct aspect of the striving, but some categories clearly overlap. Table 3.2 lists the 12 striving coding categories, with sample strivings in parentheses (see Appendix A for how to obtain the coding manual from Emmons).[1]

Starting with Achievement, we can locate Jennifer's concern with being on time as a form of achievement goal (though it clearly has affiliation and self-presentation aspects as well). Similarly, we might see her desire to do work in advance as an achievement goal, but the fact that the motive for this planning ahead is "to avoid stress" makes it seem much more like a coping goal than an achievement striving. Her overall degree of achievement content in her 13 goals is rather minimal, which fits with her low facet score on Achievement Striving for the NEO PI-R.

Moving on to Power, we are looking for evidence in Jennifer's striv-

---

TABLE 3.2. Coding Categories for Personal Strivings with Examples

1. Avoidance Goals ("to avoid risky situations")
2. Achievement ("to be successful at work")
3. Affiliation ("not to be alone")
4. Intimacy ("to be in a close loving relationship")
5. Power ("to be a leader and influence others")
6. Personal Growth and Health ("to stay fit and lose weight")
7. Self-Presentation ("to appear confident")
8. Independence ("to assert my individuality")
9. Self-Defeating ("to get on others' nerves")
10. Emotionality ("to feel things deeply and as much as possible")
11. Generativity ("to contribute to society")
12. Spirituality ("to find a deeper and spiritual meaning to life")

ing profile of a desire to influence others or make a strong impact. The only goals that could be construed as related to influencing others are two goals related to making others feel "comfortable" and "good about themselves." One might certainly see this kind of impact on others as much more about meeting their needs than about asserting one's influence over them. For this reason, Jennifer shows virtually no themes of Power, corresponding to her low level of Assertiveness on the NEO PI-R.

We can next score the two relationship motives—Affiliation and Intimacy. McAdams (1980, 1984) has spent a great deal of time distinguishing between these two motives. Affiliation is a social motive based more on the effort to achieve relationships than on enjoying their fruits. It expresses an anxious striving to avoid loneliness and to gain approval and acceptance from others (McAdams, 2006). In contrast, the Intimacy motive focuses on *being* in a relationship—the sense of closeness and warmth that individuals feel from their enjoyment of already existing connections with others. Jennifer shows Affiliation themes in her strivings to "spend as much time with my family as possible," "make others feel comfortable," and "make other people feel good about themselves." All of these strivings emphasize ways in which Jennifer can achieve positive relations with others and gain acceptance from them. They are the motivational expression of her strong Agreeableness dimension; she is highly motivated to create and maintain social environments that are familiar, comfortable, nonjudgmental, and frictionless.

In contrast, there is a virtual absence of Intimacy strivings that would convey themes of enjoying close relationships or being engaged in loving mutual interactions. Typical Intimacy strivings include "enjoy time with a close friend," "be in a sharing, loving relationship," "have good talks with someone I care about," "be a good listener," and so forth. In Jennifer, there is no sense of this relaxed or warm connection with others, especially at the one-on-one dyadic level. The combination of the Affiliation and Intimacy coding scores says much about the specific nature of Agreeableness that Jennifer expresses. The emerging picture from Domain 2 is telling us that her Agreeableness is indeed driven by her social anxiety, and not by a spontaneous and trusting warmth and engagement with other people.

Personal Growth and Health, respective to the other motives we have coded thus far, emerges with five strivings—"find ways to improve my self-esteem," "improve my personal appearance," "do my work in advance in order to avoid stress," "be open-minded about others' views," and "avoid judging others." These strivings suggest a network of expectations that Jennifer holds for herself in both the intrapersonal and interpersonal realms. Intrapersonally, she has set the goal of feeling more positively about herself, both in her thoughts and through her external appearance. She also seeks to take action that will minimize her risk of experiencing stress. Interpersonally, she has set a personal moral standard to refrain from being a narrow or judgmental person. We will need to see how effective Jennifer feels she has been so far in achieving these various goals, but, as a group, they express an acknowledgment of her frailties and limitations, as well as a determination to do better in each of these areas. It is clear that along with the regulation of her social anxiety, this domain of personal growth is very important to Jennifer, dwarfing her current concerns with either achievement or intimacy.

The link between Jennifer's Affiliative and Personal Growth motives also shows her strong concern with Self-Presentation. She wants to "avoid people who view me negatively," "to avoid seeming unintelligent," "to be on time to engagements," and "to improve my physical appearance." Not surprisingly, she shows no evidence of strivings that express her sense of Independence or Autonomy. This complete absence is more striking in consideration of Jennifer's impending graduation and the developmental demand that she assert and define herself separately from her family and others who might impinge on her emerging individuality.

The next category, Self-Defeating, is intriguing in Jennifer's case. By the coding criteria, there are no explicit statements of self-defeating or self-destructive strivings. Yet Jennifer's approach of avoiding uncomfortable situations and sticking to familiar environments seems inherently problematic for her in light of the life transition she is facing, which is filled with the prospect of novel and challenging circumstances. We do not know how her parents would receive a plan for her to move back home with them after graduation, but there may be potential tension or conflict if this is the way that she chooses to express her desire to spend as much time with them as possible.

Emotionality, the 10th coding theme, covers the degree to which Jennifer refers to the expression, understanding, and communication of emotion in any of her personal strivings. Her language about emotion in her striving list is very vague. She uses words like "uncomfortable," "stress," and "negative" rather than more specific emotion phrases like "happy," "angry," "sad," or even "anxious." There is a diffuse and pervasive interest in avoiding negative emotion states, but nothing more precise or articulated in her concern for emotion.

The last two coding themes are easily addressed. Jennifer expressed no themes of Generativity; she had no strivings related to making an artistic or social contribution to society. For example, she did not indicate that she wanted to "make the world more beautiful" or "help people in need." She also did not mention any strivings linked to Spirituality (e.g., "find a greater meaning in life," "live a religious life," or "live the way

God would want me to live"). Although one or two Generativity strivings are reasonably common among college students, it should be noted that Spirituality strivings are not as frequent. Still, her lack of these strivings is less a reflection of a negative aspect of Jennifer's profile than a statement about positive dimensions that are missing. Emmons (1999) has found that individuals with higher numbers of Generativity strivings show greater subjective well-being and satisfaction with their lives, while individuals with higher numbers of Spirituality strivings demonstrate less conflict among their various strivings. Lower conflict may indicate greater integration of the personality, which has implications for a clearer sense of meaning in life, as well as better psychological and physical health (Emmons & King, 1988).

INTERPRETING THE CONTENT
OF JENNIFER'S PERSONAL STRIVINGS

We can now step back and ask what overall conclusions we can draw from our content analysis of Jennifer's strivings. In particular, what has the striving content taught us about Jennifer above and beyond what we had learned from the NEO PI-R? First and foremost, we now see how the strivings express more clear dynamic connections among her Neuroticism, Agreeableness, Extraversion, and Conscientiousness scores. Specifically, her elevated anxiety, depression, and vulnerability to stress are linked to her strong efforts to be agreeable and lowered levels of assertiveness and angry hostility. At the same time, these elevated negative emotions reverberate with her inability to bring positive emotion into her life and her diminished sense of competence.

From her array of personal strivings, we see that Jennifer has fashioned an interpersonal world rife with the hazards of others' negative views, harsh judgments, and criticisms. Her strivings suggest that she seeks to navigate her way through this dangerous world by both limiting and controlling others' perceptions of her as much as possible. Her stated goals are to stick to the safe port of familiar and comfortable circumstances, as exemplified in the presumably nonjudgmental world of her family. However, given that this is not always possible, she will do everything in her power to manage others' impressions by appearing intelligent and attractive, and making sure that others feel comfortable and good about themselves. In her highly anxious and constricted world view, these gestures toward pleasing others are meant to neutralize the danger of being revealed for who she thinks she really is (i.e., someone who needs to improve her self-esteem, appearance, and intelligence).

Jennifer's strivings reveal just how preoccupying this struggle to regulate her stress and anxiety actually is. It leaves little room for intimacy, romance, achievement, or generative contribution to society. It forces her back to fundamental concerns of self-esteem and appearance, with little attention to goals related to enjoyment, fun, and novelty. In turn, she lacks confidence in the two primary domains that define young adult identity and growth in American culture—her achievements and relationships.

Jennifer's strivings have filled in the outline offered by her facet score of lowered competence on NEO PI-R; it is now clearer that she relates this lack of efficacy to fears about schoolwork and intelligence. Similarly, her strivings have allowed us to see that her dependency needs are focused on her family and not located for the present time in a romantic relationship. Additionally, uncertain of her own worth and highly concerned with censure by others, Jennifer is unable to assert any themes of independence or autonomy at a time period that begs for this kind of self-assertion.

This overall picture leaves us with a clearer image of Jennifer as a young woman who has not taken the formative steps in defining her own sense of self and identity. Her strivings are notable for their blandness and generality; in a literal sense, they strike one as "unformed." They are in many ways more "avoidings" than "strivings." They reflect an emotional effort of keeping one's head above a threatening sea of anxiety rather than a launching of self into the adult world.

To contrast the descriptive language of Domain 1, which portrayed Jennifer as an anxious and strongly agreeable young woman, we can now portray Jennifer as an individual striving to manage her social anxiety and struggling to stay afloat in an ominous interpersonal world. We now see that her dependency is expressed through the child-like *role* she preserves in relationship to her family as opposed to a romantic partner, that her diminished sense of competence pertains to the *contexts* of academic work and physical appearance, and that her closed approach to new ideas and experiences reflects her anxiety about being in *situations* that might expose her to criticism or ridicule. With regard to the *temporal and developmental context*, we have learned that Jennifer is facing a particular crisis by not being able to meet the autonomy and self-definition demands of identity formation in young adulthood (Erikson, 1963). The frame laid out by the NEO PI-R has now gained a more action-based orientation, along with greater contextual detail.

Yet there is still more that we can learn about Jennifer from our study of striving responses. We next turn to the analysis of the Striving Assessment Dimensions—the ratings that encompass Emmons's dimensions of Commitment/Intensity, Ease/Effort, and Desirability/Reward. These ratings show us how Jennifer prioritizes her various strivings and her sense of efficacy in reaching the goals she sets for herself.

INTERPRETING THE STRIVING DIMENSIONS

Looking across each row in Table 3.3 allows us to see how desirable each striving is, how committed Jennifer is to the pursuit of that striving, and the degree of difficulty she associates with its attainment. Looking down the column gives a sense of how each of these three features applies in general across the 13 strivings in Jennifer's life. To explore Desirability/Reward, we selected three Dimension Scales: (1) How Much Happiness Attainment of the Striving Would Bring; (2) How Much *Un*happiness Nonattainment of the Striving Would Bring; and (3) Ambivalence about Attainment. To explore Commitment/Intensity, we selected (4) Commitment to Attainment. To explore Ease/Effort, we selected (5) Success in the Past Month and (6) Probability of Future Success.

Desirability–Reward

As we can see in looking at the first column, 9 of the 13 strivings received scores of *very much* or *much happiness* upon attainment, though, interestingly, no striving received a top score of 5 or *extreme happiness*. The three that would bring *very much happiness* are "spending time with my family," "improving self-esteem," and "improving my appearance." The four that would bring only *moderate happiness* (score of 2) are "doing work in advance," "being open-minded," "remaining in a familiar environment," and "being on time to engagements." With the exception of open-mindedness, the other three seem to be anxiety-management strategies; therefore, it is easy to see why they bring only moderate levels of happiness by their attainment.

Turning to the Unhappiness category, looking down the column, we can see that there is much more variability in what would bring Jennifer unhappiness on nonattainment. Interestingly, only two strivings would bring only slight unhappiness if not attained—"remaining in a familiar environment," and "being on time to engagements." Since these two would also bring only moderate happiness on attainment, we can see them as lower level strivings in terms of how much passion they generate in Jennifer. There are six strivings that would generate moderate amounts of unhappiness if nonattained. More importantly, there are five strivings that would lead to *much* to *extreme* degrees of unhappiness by their nonattainment. To begin, the two rat-

TABLE 3.3. Jennifer's Striving Assessment Matrix

Strivings	Happiness	Unhappiness	Ambivalence	Commitment	Past attainment	Probability of success
1. Avoid uncomfortable situations.	3	2	2	3	7	7
2. Make others feel comfortable.	3	2	1	4	8	8
3. Spend time with my family.	4	4	0	5	9	8
4. Improve my self-esteem.	4	5	0	4	2	3
5. Do work to avoid stress.	2	2	1	3	7	6
6. Make others feel good.	3	2	0	3	6	7
7. Be open-minded.	2	2	1	4	7	7
8. Avoid people who view me negatively.	3	3	1	3	7	7
9. Improve my appearance.	4	4	0	4	3	5
10. Remain in a familiar environment.	2	1	2	2	6	6
11. Be on time to my engagements.	2	1	0	3	8	8
12. Avoid seeming unintelligent.	3	3	1	3	4	5
13. Avoid judging others.	3	2	1	3	7	6
Rating scale	0–5 5: Extreme happiness	0–5 5: Extreme unhappiness	0–5 5: Very much unhappiness	0–5 5: Extremely committed	0–9 0: 0–9% 9: 90–100%	0–9 0: 0–9% 9–90%

61

ings of *much* (3) were for "avoiding people who view me negatively" and "avoiding seeming unintelligent." Once again, exposure to individuals' negative judgment is a central concern, and not meeting these goals opens up a potential flood of criticism and imagined ridicule. The two strivings that received 4's, meaning *very much unhappiness*, were "spending time with my family" and "improving my appearance"; Jennifer is once again consistent in placing these concerns as critical to her emotional equilibrium. At the highest level, and the only striving to receive a 5 for *extreme unhappiness* if not attained, is "improving my self-esteem." It would seem that many of the other strivings are encapsulated in this fundamental self-doubt that nags Jennifer and organizes much of her social behavior.

We can next look at Jennifer's Ambivalence on attaining a striving. For 11 of 13 strivings, she indicates that she would feel *no* or *very slight unhappiness* on their attainment, suggesting that she is clear on her commitment to these goal pursuits. However, two strivings yielded scores of *slight unhappiness* on attainment—"avoiding uncomfortable situations" and "remaining in familiar situations." Clearly, Jennifer senses that there are costs to avoiding any novelty or challenge in her life. She may indeed see that her social anxiety closes doors for her and does not allow her as much freedom as she might ideally like.

Commitment

Regarding her level of Commitment to her strivings, Jennifer indicated moderate to strong commitment for 12 of 13 strivings. The only striving that received a lower level of commitment was "remaining in familiar situations," which fits the pattern of ambivalence she has thus far displayed toward this striving. The striving of "spending time with family" was the only one to receive a 5, indicating the greatest possible commitment.

Difficulty–Ease

The final two dimensions provide insight into the past difficulty and future probability of attainment that Jennifer associates with each striving. In the past month, she felt that she has been 90–100% successful in only one striving—"spending time with family." She has been 80–89% successful in two others—"making others feel comfortable" and "being on time to engagements." She assigned a 70–79% success rate to five strivings—"avoiding uncomfortable situations," "doing work in advance to avoid stress," "avoiding people who view me negatively," "avoiding judging others," and "being open-minded." She has been 60–

69% successful in two more—"making others feel good about themselves" and "remaining in a familiar environment."

This total leaves three critical strivings for which Jennifer perceives her success rate to be only 50–59% or lower. First, she sees herself as only 40–49% successful in "avoiding seeming unintelligent." She sees herself as only 30–39% successful in "improving my physical appearance." Finally, she sees herself as only 20–29% successful in "improving my self-esteem." In these critical strivings that focus on personal growth, health, and self-presentation, Jennifer sees herself as currently falling powerfully short of her desired aims. Combined with the fact that she has rated these particular goals as ones that bring her relatively more happiness on attainment and greater unhappiness on nonattainment, we see the emergence of what Higgins (1987) would call a high level of "self-discrepancy." Jennifer's actual self, as she perceives it, is falling far short of her ideal or desired self in these critical areas of personal esteem and self-confidence. Higgins has demonstrated repeatedly that high self-discrepancies are related to vulnerability to depression and anxiety disorders.

To finish Table 3.3, we can look at how Jennifer estimates her rates of success for the future. In a positive light, she does estimate that she will do 70% or better in attaining seven (or more than half) of her strivings. Once again, these successes tend to focus on her avoidance goals and capacity to make others feel comfortable. She sees herself only slightly less successful on three strivings (60–69%)—"doing work in advance," "being on time to engagements," and "avoiding judging others." Yet the two goals for which she sees only a 50–59% chance for success in the future are "improving my appearance" and "avoiding seeming unintelligent." Finally, she estimates only a 30–39% chance of "improving my self-esteem," once again giving the greatest difficulty score to the striving that she also rated as likely to bring her the most unhappiness if not attained.

In looking at the last two columns in Table 3.3, it is useful to note increases or decreases from past to future. For example, Jennifer sees herself as just a bit less likely to succeed in the future in "spending time with my family." Perhaps her senior year in college has influenced this prediction. She does see the prospects for "improving my self-esteem" as rising slightly, which is an encouraging sign. She sees her possibility of "avoiding work stress" as worsening but envisions better prospects for "making others feel good about themselves," "improving my physical appearance," and "avoiding feeling unintelligent." Last, she sees her chances of "avoiding judging others" as slightly declining, which might actually be a positive if it suggests Jennifer's increased willingness to assert her own opinions.

OVERALL INTERPRETATION OF
STRIVING ASSESSMENT DIMENSIONS

The analysis of the striving assessment dimensions has added a sense of dynamics and motion to our coding of striving content. The dimensions make clear that Jennifer's greatest area of focus is protecting and enhancing her self-esteem, while at the same time staying close to her family. We see from the dimensions of Commitment and Reward how determined she is to feel better about herself and to avoid negative evaluations, but we also see her estimates of how successful she has been and will be in these efforts. Fitting with her concerns about competence and her strong tendency toward negative emotion, we see that she views her progress in the critical goals of feeling more intelligent and attractive as still not reaching much beyond a 50% success rate. Also, aligned with her low Positive Emotions score on the Extraversion dimension of the NEO PI-R, we see that Jennifer does not imagine that success in any striving will bring her extreme happiness. On the other hand, she readily acknowledges that failing to improve her self-esteem brings her extreme unhappiness.

The dimensional analysis also further confirms our sense that Jennifer's interpersonal world is more focused on regulating potential negative outcomes than on taking real pleasure in connections with others. Though pleasing others brings her much happiness, she reserves her highest ratings for improving her appearance and self-esteem. The one exception is how much pleasure she takes in time spent with her family. She may indeed feel safest and most comfortable in her home environment, yet her predictions about the future indicate that her opportunity to have the safety and warmth of home may soon diminish.

There is even more that could be done with Jennifer's dimensional ratings by considering them in comparison to those of other college students who have completed the same dimensional matrix for their strivings. We could see how her average happiness ratings or past attainment estimates compare to other students who might bring a more optimistic or positive emotion outlook to their striving attainment efforts (Emmons, 1999, provides some of this helpful nomothetic information). For now, we might simply note that Jennifer's process of striving attainment—how she values her strivings, commits to them, and expends effort on their behalf—continues to reflect the profile of someone who is suffering from a combination of low self-esteem, anxious depression, and a clear dependence on her family to help her regulate her social anxiety. We see increasingly that her psychological world is dominated by these worries and insecurities at the expense of making intimate connections with others outside her family, as well as setting limits on the genuine pleasure she takes in her successes and interactions with others.

Having identified these core areas of concern for Jennifer, we turn to consideration of how she manages to adjust to social demands and to defend against the outbreak of distress and helpless frustration in her life. In other words, to fill in another dimension of what is still missing from a comprehensive understanding of Jennifer, we still need to know how Jennifer negotiates her way through daily life. What mechanisms of self-restraint and defense does she employ to modulate her anxiety and avoid succumbing to her depression? These questions once again reflect a Domain 2 analysis that asks how individuals cope with the various situations in which they find themselves at different developmental periods in their lives. To address these issues of adjustment and defense, we selected a relatively brief but powerfully informative instrument, the Weinberger Adjustment Inventory—Short Form (Weinberger, 1997, 1998).

ADJUSTMENT AND DEFENSES

By examining the dynamic quality of Jennifer's strivings, we have already hinted at how we might understand her effort to control negative emotion and avoid feelings of criticism and inferiority in her life. Weinberger (1998, p. 1062) defined *defense mechanisms* as "a set of mediating *processes* that buffer perceptions of internal or external threat [emphasis in original]." Dating back to Freud's (1915/1953) original ideas on the unconscious and his daughter Anna's (1936) elaboration of types of defense, a consistent line of theory and research has focused on how individuals protect themselves from negative evaluation and regulate their affective experiences. As Anna Freud suggested, much of this research has conceptualized defenses along a continuum associated with the maturity of ego development. The types of defenses one employs are associated with one's capacity to control impulses, take planful action, tolerate ambiguity, and negotiate nuanced interpersonal relationships (Loevinger, 1976, 1983).

Westen (1998), in his overview of Freud's scientific legacy, has reviewed the empirical evidence for this position. For example, he describes the work of Vaillant (Vaillant, 1977, 1992; Vaillant & McCullough, 1998), which has demonstrated that one can reliably identify four levels of defenses at increasing levels of maturity, ranging from flagrant denial of reality at the lowest level to the subtle use of humor and appropriate sublimation at the highest level. By collecting longitudinal samples, Vaillant has consistently shown that individuals' characteristic levels of defenses are associated over time with both psychological health and proneness to personality disorders (Vaillant & Drake, 1985).

Westen (1998) also reviewed his own classification of defenses, developed from a Q-sort and factor-analytic procedure based on clinical descriptions of 90 patients (Westen, Muderrisoglu, Fowler, Shedler, & Koren, 1997). This work identified three dimensions of defense. He called the first "adaptive regulation," which consists of "active coping versus acting impulsively." Active copers approach problems through planning, information gathering, and problem solving. Impulsive actors engage in denial, acting out, and substance abuse. The second factor, "externalizing defenses," consists of two poles of "blaming others versus blaming the self." Blaming others is associated with a refusal to accept responsibility for one's difficulties, and unrealistic self-promotion and the inflation of one's successes. In contrast, blaming the self reflects a tendency to avoid expression of anger at others' actions and a reversal of that anger on to the self, resulting in self-derogation and passivity. The third factor, "avoidant defenses," identified individuals' tendency to push negative affect out of awareness versus a preoccupation with the experience and expression of negative affect. Individuals high in affect avoidance tend toward intellectualization and repression of any unpleasant affect, while individuals at the other pole ruminate over their distress, veer back and forth between seeking comfort from and avoiding others, and often display physical symptoms related to their distress. Similar to Vaillant, Westen (1991) demonstrated that poor object relations and more extreme forms of defense, such as splitting and rapid shifts in idealization and devaluation, as measured through TAT protocols, were associated with the more severe pathology of borderline and narcissistic personality disorders.

Importantly, other researchers, Cramer (Sandstrom & Cramer, 2003a, 2003b) and Bandura, Barbarnelli, Caprara, and Pastorelli (1996), have demonstrated that defensive variations in children are associated with their relative levels of maturity and the quality of their peer relations. For example, Sandstrom and Cramer (2003b) found that elementary school girls who displayed more basic and child-like defenses of denial and aggression on TAT protocols were more likely to receive rejection from peers than those children who employed more sophisticated defenses of sublimation and reframing of negative experiences.

Weinberger (1997, 1998) argued that a common threat in all these theories of defenses as a form of personality development is that defenses emerge from the appropriate application of self-control to desires and impulses, as well as the regulation of affect. As individuals participate first in family relationships, and increasingly in social interactions and various communities and institutions outside the family, the need to modulate urges, emotional displays, and behavior becomes a fundamental requirement of maturity and effective human functioning. Censure, punishment, shame, and, eventually, internalized guilt all serve to invoke anxiety in the face of "antisocial" expressions of wishes or affects. Since restraint of needs and urges is inherently frustrating, but their expression can provoke an even more powerful distress, we develop defenses to manage the tension between release and control of our desires. Weinberger (1998) wrote:

> For Freud, the quintessential dilemma of human existence is the inherent conflict between the desire to avoid distress by focusing on one's own immediate gratification versus the need to assimilate the constraints imposed by others and the reality principle. . . . Hence an important aspect of personality structure can be defined in terms of the general level of *self-restraint* individuals exhibit in conjunction with their subjective *distress* about their concomitant ability to meet their own needs. . . . (p. 1065; emphasis in original)

Weinberger Adjustment Inventory—Short Form

Out of this formulation of defense and personality structure, Weinberger (1995, 1997, 1998; Weinberger & Schwartz, 1990) developed the Weinberger Adjustment Inventory (WAI) to capture how individuals regulate these two dimensions of Self-Restraint and Distress. This inventory consists of 84 items with four subscales for Self-Restraint—self-control (Impulse Control), interpersonal control (Suppression of Aggression; Consideration of Others), and social restraint (Responsibility)—and four subscales for Distress—proneness to negative affect (Anxiety; Depression), lack of positive affect (Low Well-Being), and negative affect turned on the self (Low Self-Esteem), along with a subscale for denial of distress and one for repressive defensiveness. The Weinberger Adjustment Inventory—Short Form (WAI-SF) consists of 37 items, the four subscales for Self-Restraint and the four for Distress, along with the Repressive Defensiveness subscale. Each item uses a 1- to 5-point Likert-type scale, with 1 indicating False (*almost never*) and 5, True (*almost always*). In order to counteract response sets and disguise social desirability, there are many reversed items.

Low restraint scores are characteristic of young children or individuals who do not regulate their impulses and affects successfully, and are associated with problem behavior such as drug use, delinquency, and aggression (for summaries, see Farrell & Sullivan, 2000; Weinberger,

1998). Excessive self-restraint is the result of socialization and can be considered more adaptive; however, individuals who are best adapted socially and emotionally should show moderate self-restraint as they manage affect skillfully and do not become rigid or overly intellectualized (Asendorpf & van Aken, 1999; Hart, Hofmann, Edelstein, & Keller, 1997; Weinberger & Schwartz, 1990). The Subjective Experience of Distress captures the self's own appraisal of its status in relation to personal goals, as well as to external sources of threat. Weinberger (1995, 1997) has provided validation of the Distress dimension, as have independent researchers (e.g., Garner, Steiner, Huckaby, & Kohler, 1998).

The Repressive Defensiveness scale measures individuals' tendencies to avoid negative evaluation and promote a positive self-presentation, independent of actual levels of distress (Weinberger & Davidson, 1994). Turvey and Salovey (1993–1994) compared it to four other previous defensiveness and repression scales, and found it to be superior in terms of internal consistency, normal distribution, and efficiency to administer.

Table 3.4 presents each of the subscales for the two dimensions of Self-Restraint and Distress, as well as for Repressive Defensiveness, along with representative items. For the first two dimensions, each subscale consists of three items apiece, combining for 12 items for each dimension. The Repressive Defensiveness scale has 11 items and has two

TABLE 3.4. Weinberger Adjustment Inventory—Short Form (WAI-SF): Subscales and Representative Items

Self-Restraint
1. Impulse Control (I do things without giving them enough thought.—Reversed)
2. Supression of Aggression (I can remember a time when I was so angry at someone that I felt like hurting them.—Reversed)
3. Consideration of Others (Before I do something, I think about how it will affect the people around me.)
4. Responsibility (I do things that I know really aren't right.—Reversed)

Distress
1. Anxiety (I worry too much about things that aren't important.)
2. Depression (I often feel sad or unhappy.)
3. Low Self-Esteem (I really don't like myself very much.)
4. Low Well-Being (I usually think of myself as a happy person.—Reversed)

Repressive Defensiveness
1. I never act like I know more about something than I really do.
2. Once in a while, I break a promise I've made.—Reversed

validity items (e.g., "I am answering these questions truthfully"). For information on how to obtain the short form or the full inventory, as well as detailed scoring instructions, please see Appendix A, this volume.

Scoring the WAI-SF

To score the WAI-SF, we calculated the scores for each subscale within each dimension (being careful to reverse values for reversed items) and then totaled the subscales, yielding overall Self-Restraint and overall Distress scores. We then summed the 11 Repressive Defensiveness items (once again taking into account reversed items) to obtain that overall score. With tables supplied by Weinberger (personal e-mail communication, March 2002), we located where Jennifer placed in relationship to other college students. On the dimension of Self-Restraint, her overall score was 52, which means that she averaged 4.33 out of 5 or more than *somewhat true* in responding to items involving self-control and suppression of her impulses. Compared to her peers, she scored in the 80–90% range for Self-Restraint.

For the dimension of Distress, she scored a total of 46, averaging 3.83 or just under *somewhat true* for items indicating a general unhappiness and dissatisfaction with the self. This total placed her in the highest 95–100% of her peers, indicating an extreme degree of Distress.

Finally, her Repressive Defensiveness total was 43, averaging 3.9 or essentially *somewhat true* for items related to her tendency to present herself in the most positive light and to deny any negative conduct. Her high Repressive Defensiveness score once again placed her in the 95–100% bracket compared to her peers.

Interpreting Scores on the WAI-SF

Weinberger (1998) has defined six typologies that emerge from the combination of the Self-Restraint and Distress dimensions. He created these six groups by dividing Self-Restraint scores into three categories—low, moderate, and high (the numerical values for each category depends on the peer comparison)—and the Distress scores into two categories—low and high. He has found that the division of Self-Restraint into three groups is optimal in order to distinguish between individuals who show a well-modulated control and those who are impulsive on the one hand and too rigidly or tightly controlled on the other. For Distress, two categories appear to be most effective, because efforts to distinguish between low and moderate distress runs into the problem of distinguishing truly low distress individuals from those who may be employing some degree of defensiveness. Empirically, he has found that two categories of high and low produce the most reliable and accurate differentiation of Distress in a given sample of participants.

The six groups, defined by Weinberger (1998, p. 1066), are

- Low Distress/Low Self-Restraint (Undersocialized)
- High Distress/Low Self-Restraint (Reactive)
- Low Distress/Moderate Self-Restraint (Self-Assured)
- High Distress/Moderate Self-Restraint (Sensitized)
- Low Distress/High Self-Restraint (Repressive)
- High Distress/High Self-Restraint (Oversocialized)

Based on her scores, Jennifer belongs in the Oversocialized group. According to Weinberger (1998), this category suggests that Jennifer is uncomfortable with putting her needs before those of others. She is likely to be prone to guilt and social anxiety. Most importantly, with regard to her defenses, she is highly protected against any form of threat and relies on more primitive strategies of denial, minimization, and reaction formation. To avoid conflict over impulse expression, she adheres to a conventional pattern of behavior that places her at the conformist or "interpersonal" stage of ego development (Kegan, 1982; Loevinger, 1976; see Weinberger, 1998, p. 1074). Her superego, or moral standard, is not fully internalized; she is still highly influenced by important others, especially authority figures, in her moral decisions and choices. Her attachment style, as conceptualized by Bartholomew and Horowitz (1991), is "Fearful," meaning she struggles to communicate her desires in relationships and may even avoid relationships due to anxiety about rejection. Interestingly, Weinberger (1998, p. 1075) points to research that particularly identifies this attachment style with restricting female anorexics (Steiner & Feldman, 1995).

OVERALL INTERPRETATION OF
WAIS-SF AND STRIVINGS TOGETHER

The WAIS-SF, as developed by Weinberger, offers a different but converging perspective with the personal striving analysis of Domain 2. His blend of psychoanalytic and social-cognitive frameworks portrays personality as developing from the efforts to negotiate the inevitable conflict of desires and social relations with others. How individuals use defenses to manage this tension, along with resultant affective responses, reflects their relative levels of maturity and ego development. Jennifer's rigid and fearful self-restraint, combined with her inability to moderate her negative feelings of depression, anxiety, and guilt, suggest that she is still relatively unsophisticated in her defensive structure and ego maturity.

We could indeed conceptualize some of her NEO PI-R facet scores as reflecting these defensive dynamics. For example, Jennifer's markedly low score on Angry Hostility, in contrast to several elevated Neuroticism facets, now makes even more sense. She may indeed deny hostility or use reaction formation to turn her anger at others onto herself. This tendency corresponds to Westen's (Westen et al., 1997) pole of "blaming the self" in his "externalizing defenses" dimension. Similarly, her high level of Agreeableness and low Assertiveness may reflect an "undoing" style of defense in which she excessively tries to please others to make up for self-perceived inadequacy or momentary lapses of impulsive behavior (see Weinberger, 1998, p. 1074). Her high level of Repressive Defensiveness additionally indicates an intense concern with self-presentation and a great difficulty acknowledging any kind of socially inappropriate or impulse-gratifying behavior. The combination of these oversocialized defenses is indeed associated with disorders focused on excessive restraint and battles with impulse expression, most notably eating and obsessive–compulsive disorders.

Our understanding of Jennifer has again advanced to give us a sense of her psychological dynamics and how they are expressed in her efforts to manage her relations with others, as well as her own emotions. Analysis of her strivings and her defenses has yielded a picture of a young woman who in many ways is resisting a transition to adulthood. Fearful of judgment and criticism from others, she is strongly wedded to her family and inhibited in her emotional expression and action. To manage her anxiety about others and her own emotions, she relies heavily on controlling her self-presentation, both physically and intellectually. These efforts reduce her opportunity for spontaneous pleasure and limit her capacity to develop more in-depth relationships outside her family. Her preoccupation with her own emotional world and personal health has hindered her ability to connect to a larger world beyond herself and to express goals or ambitions beyond her immediate defensive stance. Her strong defensiveness is likely to take rather immature forms, which include turning her frustration with others onto her self and excessively overcompensating for any momentary lapses that she perceives in her strong efforts at self-control. In its most dangerous form, the combination of poor self-image and rigid controls on her self-expression and desires might point to a range of disorders related to struggles over impulse management, including possible obsessive–compulsive or eating disorder difficulties.

WHAT IS MISSING?

Indulging for a moment in a detective metaphor, thus far we have followed the trail of Jennifer's personality in the dark. She initially entered our office, asked for our help, filled out our questionnaires, and then disappeared. What we know of Jennifer is based only in these psychometric tests, the barest demographic details, and a brief glimpse of her physical appearance. Our chain of inferences is like one woven by Sam Spade or Sherlock Holmes from a lock of hair left behind or a smell of a rare perfume that persists in an abandoned room. We can develop an increasingly rich and compelling story, but it will always be missing two ingredients. In a sense, these two ingredients pull us in opposite directions—one toward the darkness, and the other more blatantly into the light.

First, the darkness: What more might we learn of aspects of Jennifer's personality that are hidden from her own conscious awareness? Are there ambivalences toward her family, sexual desires, and aggressive impulses that she has pushed aside or buried that help to explain the depth of her anxiety and the strength of her defenses? By employing two self-report questionnaires (the NEO PI-R and the WAI-SF) and one semistructured measure (Personal Strivings), we have had little opportunity to tap into these potential unconscious influences. It is indeed intriguing to consider whether projective measures such as the Rorschach test or the TAT, would allow us to access a further level of depth. As I mentioned in the Introduction to this volume, much of the 20th-century linkage between personality and psychotherapy was based on these two personality assessment tests. Behrends and Blatt (2003) amply demonstrate how complex and subtle an interpretation of personality these measures can provide. Yet once again, my goal in this volume is to introduce newer personality assessment instruments to a wide range of students and therapists, many of whom might not subscribe to a psychoanalytic perspective. The cost of this decision may be that I continue to leave some readers asking for more, frustrated that the wholeness of Jennifer has not been grasped. I can only agree and encourage all students of personality and therapists, when possible, to apply projective instruments that may allow one to go deeper and to look harder for what may be there at another level of illumination. Yet this volume's task thus far has set a different priority—the explication of three domains of personality through the lens of innovative, newer methods of personality research. In Chapter 5, as I address what is still missing from this three-domain framework, we return to this problem of unconscious processes and more squarely examine some of these issues by looking at the phenomenon of intersubjectivity in psychotherapy. With regard to Jennifer, there may indeed be darker sides to her nature that our current inquiry ultimately has failed to tap. Granting this limitation, I return to the question of what remains to be elucidated within our current framework by our final set of investigative methods.

We are about to view Jennifer in the light of her life history and to learn from her what she sees as the critical events that give meaning and definition to her sense of self. In the parlance of the detective and police world, we need to "identify" the missing person. As indicated in the Introduction of this volume, *identity* is the means by which individuals form a coherent self-narrative that links past, present, and future into a meaningful whole. It is also the manner in which they take the demographic features of their life—their gender, ethnicity, religion, class, sexuality—and connect them to the larger social and cultural worlds that they inhabit. On these and other self-defining dimensions, where does Jennifer see herself as fitting in (or not fitting in) with the world of adults that she has so recently joined?

In asking these questions, we can finally bring the search for Jennifer back to the most familiar realm of how we know another person. We can learn from her own words about her life details; we can hear directly about the events she sees as pivotal for her and the meanings she attaches to them. We can begin to glean how she constructs her current sense of self in light of the apparent struggles she has had with her anxieties and insecurities. We might also be able to discern more clearly the areas of strengths she possesses, as well as additional resources that she does not reveal in her often harsh self-assessments.

Most of all, it is time to learn Jennifer's story—how she assembles the specific events of her life that have been experienced by no one else in the unique way that she has lived them, and turns these moments and episodes into an overarching self-narrative. By collecting her self-defining memories and life history, we will begin to hear the beating heart beneath the powerful frame of flesh and bone we have thus far assembled.

NOTE

1. In coding for these themes, it should be noted that there is a substantial theoretical and research literature on what it means to code for these motivational themes using more conscious measures of personality. Various personality researchers have attempted to flesh out the different aspects of social motives that conscious measures (e.g., self-report questionnaires of motivation) and

more unconscious methods (e.g., TAT) assess (Koestner, Weinberger, & McClelland, 1991; McClelland, Koestner, & Weinberger, 1989; Schultheiss & Brunstein, 1999). These authors have indicated that conscious measures are more likely to tap into *explicit or self-attributed motives*, which are more dictated by a particular context or situation, and the expectations associated with that context. In contrast, unconscious techniques access *implicit motives*, which predict less context-sensitive and more long-term patterns of desire and behavior.

For example, explicit measures of motives are reasonably effective at predicting individuals' achievement or affiliation behavior in situations that pull for these motives, respectively. For example, a self-report measure that captures an individual's level of achievement motivation will provide a good read on that person's likelihood to exert effort in a competitive game or academic examination. In contrast, social motives measured by the TAT are more effective in predicting individuals' thoughts and behaviors in more open situations, where demands for achievement or affiliation are less clearly specified. A high need for achievement score on a TAT protocol might predict that an individual would end up playing competitive board games during a ski weekend. Perhaps this latter more unstructured situation gives more opportunity for the latent and unique themes of the individual personality to emerge. In a sense, these less defined contexts are similar to the experience afforded by the TAT cards themselves, which, by their ambiguous qualities, encourage individuals to project their more latent personal themes on to the card images.

If this analysis is accurate, then trait measures or personality inventories that explicitly measure motives (e.g., Jackson Personality Research Form, PRF; Jackson, 1974) might identify individuals' overt or self-presentational responses to situational demands, while TAT measurements would reveal their more intrinsic and self-initiated motive concerns. Researchers who have employed questionnaire measures that tap achievement, power, or intimacy motives, along with TAT protocols in the same study, have found very little correlation between the two different indices of the same motives (Entwisle, 1972; King, 1995; McClelland, 1985).

Turning to our current work, where would personal strivings fit in this debate? Given that the personal striving technique is not only conscious but also open-ended, it should fall in the middle, between the two explicit and implicit motive techniques; that is, the personal striving task does tap into the self-attribution process, since individuals are not projecting potentially unconscious themes on to the fantasy stories of the TAT. Rather, they are consciously identifying what they typically want to do in their lives. On the other hand, because they are answering this question to an open-ended stem (i.e., "I typically try to. . ."), they are able to respond in an idiographic manner that allows for the expression of their more personal, enduring, and decontextualized concerns. In this manner, personal strivings are once again a "middle-level" construct of motivation—hovering between explicit and implicit motives.

To demonstrate this position empirically, Emmons and McAdams (1991) found moderate correlations between TAT scoring for motives of achievement, power and intimacy, and motive coding of personal strivings. This finding suggests that the coding of social motives for personal strivings allows us to access at least some aspects of both individuals' context-dependent motivational responses and their more long-term intrinsic personal motives.

4

Domain 3—
Narrative Identity

Life Stories and Self-Defining Memories

Behavioral observation is . . . inferior to the personal document
when it comes to the important region of subjective meaning:
experiences of love, beauty, [and] religious faith; of pain,
ambition, fear, jealousy, [and] frustration, plans, remembrances,
fantasies, and friendships; none of these topics come fully within
the horizon of psychologists without the aid of personal
reporting. If these regions of experience are excluded, mental
science finds itself confined to a shadowy subject matter.
                    —ALLPORT (1942, cited in Wertz, 2001, p. 237)

One of the more unusual plays to appear on Broadway in the
last several years was a one-actor play, *I Am My Own Wife*, written by
Doug Wright. In the play, the actor Jefferson Mays portrays Charlotte
von Mahlsdorf (born Lothar Berfelde), a German curio collector who
died in 2002 at 74. Charlotte, who was born a male but identified as a
female, lived through the successive brutal treatment of first the Nazis
and then the Stasi, the East German secret police. In order to convey
Charlotte's story, Mays slips periodically out of his characterization of
Charlotte to inhabit 34 other characters who intersected at different
points with Charlotte's life. As if this complexity were not enough, one
of these characters is the playwright Wright himself, who is attempting
to discern the true from the distorted memories that Charlotte has assembled in her life story. Ultimately, the play is as much about the nature

of memory and how one constructs a narrative of self as it is a testament
to Charlotte's uncanny ability to survive. In his review of the play, *The
New York Times* critic Bruce Weber wrote:

> Ah, but are [her memories] credible? That becomes an issue in the play,
> which very subtly but in the end quite powerfully makes a case for the
> necessity of storytelling in our lives. Among the resonant assertions of "I
> Am My Own Wife" is that lives themselves are narratives, and that the
> perspective, sympathy, and reliability of the narrator are crucial to our
> understanding of them. ("Inventing her Life as She Goes Along,"
> nytimes.com/2003/12/04/arts/theater/04wife.html?8hpib, p. 2)

Ultimately, for one's sense of self or narrative identity, the truth of
the memories one recalls is less critical than their linkage to one's most
important goals and desires. As Alfred Adler (1927, 1930) expressed at
the beginning of the previous century, our memories are projections of
our most enduring goals and attitudes; they represent not so much a
veridical account of the past as a revealing window into what matters to
us now; that is, he believed that one's earliest memory would reveal less
about the effect of that experience on one's subsequent life than it might
about how one had infused the memory with pressing desires of the moment. If this is the case, then to study how individuals tell the stories of
their lives, or to collect their most significant memories, is simultaneously to learn of their past and their present. In this chapter, asking
Jennifer to provide a general narrative of her life, as well as memories of
specific, self-defining moments, should uncover critical aspects of her
current sense of identity.

Identity, as Erikson (1959, 1963; see also McAdams, 2006, pp. 352–
359) first defined the concept, is a fundamental answer to the questions,
"Who am I?" and "Where do I fit in adult society?" He suggested that
individuals engage in a form of "triple-bookkeeping" that attempts to
reconcile biological, psychological, and social/interpersonal demands on
the self. To construct a sense of identity is to assert a set of beliefs, values, and goals that expresses the potentials and limits of the body, mind,
and culture that comprise the full extent of one's life. Successful identity
construction leads to a sense of integration or unity and a conviction
that one's life matters and is purposeful not only to oneself but also to
intimate others, and to the larger communities of friendship, work, and
faith that make up the social fabric.

Building on Freud's psychosexual stages of development, Erikson
(1963) proposed that individuals move through eight stages of the human life cycle, with each stage defined by a critical developmental challenge. I have listed these in Table 4.1, since they form a critical backdrop

TABLE 4.1. Erikson's Eight Psychosocial Stages of Life

1. Infancy (approximately 0–2 years)—trust versus mistrust
2. Early childhood (approximately 2–3 years)—autonomy versus shame and doubt
3. Childhood (approximately 3–5 years)—initiative versus guilt
4. School age (approximately 5–12 years)—industry versus inferiority
5. Adolescence and young adult (approximately 12–22 years)—identity versus role confusion
6. Young adult (approximately 20s and 30s)—intimacy versus isolation
7. Mid-adulthood (approximately 30s–60s)—generativity versus stagnation
8. Old age (approximately 60s–D)—ego integrity versus despair

for consideration of the life story of identity that Jennifer will be asked to tell. At the first stage, infants are preoccupied by basic needs that must be met by others who provide nurturance and security. Depending on the reliability of caretakers, they develop a benevolent and trusting view of the world or else learn to fear that others will not be able to meet their needs.

As children develop control of their own bodies, their concern shifts from dependence to an emerging independence and self-mastery. This second stage is typified by efforts to master toilet training, as well as toddlers' first concerted efforts at walking and manipulating objects in the service of their goals and desires. Success in these activities leads to a sense of autonomy and self-confidence, while struggles with self-assertion lead to humiliation, shame, and embarrassment.

The third stage of early childhood (initiative vs. guilt) parallels Freud's psychosexual Oedipal stage. In this period, children begin to grasp the potential power that autonomy provides. Propelled by a naive egocentrism, they express grandiose and at times aggressive wishes, and press others to conform to their desires (the most grandiose, of course, is Freud's controversial notion of the wish to supplant their same-sex parent and become the partner to their respective opposite-sex parent). The benefits of this initiative stage are dramatic leaps forward in mastery of various developmental challenges (e.g., dressing themselves, acquiring information, learning social cues), but the risk is that their self-assertion can hurt or trouble others, resulting in a sense of guilt and remorse. If this stage is not successfully resolved, individuals may have later difficulty with taking independent action and negotiating how to assert their wishes appropriately in relationships with others.

Moving on from early childhood, Erikson saw the socialization processes of peer relationships and school life as increasingly dominating individuals' development in the fourth stage. Fitting into the world outside the family requires an increasing mastery of skills, tools, and roles that allow for successful participation in contemporary society. The "industrious" children of today learn to read and write, tell time, use a computer, operate the microwave, and work the cell phone. Along the way, they might also learn to ride a bicycle, dribble a soccer ball, and play an instrument. Simultaneously, children are learning rules of conduct and morality—what to value and what to discount. They are incorporating the cultural histories and standards of their communities and their nations, which can provide further sources of pride or inferiority. As the needs of the body tend to dominate the earlier stages of development, the demands of "fitting in" and finding a place among one's peers now takes a central place in the life cycle.

With the emergence of adolescence, individuals have gone through biological and cognitive changes that prepare them for entry into the adult world. Cognitively, their capacity for formal operations (Inhelder & Piaget, 1958) allows them to step out of their own lives and contemplate abstract worlds or possibilities. They are increasingly able to imagine ideal worlds that can be held up as models to work for or urge others to embrace. They can project themselves forward into possible careers, relationships, and lifestyles, imagining what the pleasures or limitations of these choices might be. Similarly, they can begin to look back and reflect on their own personal histories, seeing influences and incidents that have helped to shape their current personality. In Erikson's fifth stage, both processes of looking back and looking forward are expressions of the adolescent's fundamental efforts to answer the question "Who am I?"

Since Erikson, identity researchers (e.g., Marcia, 1980; Waterman, 1982) have looked at the process of commitment that adolescents and young adults make to occupational and ideological positions that express their emerging self-definitions. Depending on the degree of active exploration and resolution in which they engage, individuals can be assigned to one of four statuses. If individuals adopt an active, challenging stance to parental values and societal norms, but do not yet commit to their own distinct values and beliefs, then they are considered to be in a *moratorium* status. Individuals who move from the moratorium status to a state of commitment are deemed *identity achieved*. Those individuals who simply adopt the existing values of family and society, without a period of active questioning, belong to a *foreclosed* status, while those who neither explore nor commit, but simply drift and avoid the demands of adulthood, fill the last category of *identity diffused*.

In a longitudinal study of women classified in one of the four statuses during their senior college year, Josselson (1996) found that this last category of "drifters" was the slowest of the four groups to reach an articulated direction in their lives, but that they did grow ultimately more introspective and gain greater control over their lives as they entered their 30s and 40s. Still, their desultory pace led to several regrets about missed opportunities and often a sense of midlife crisis at the prospect of their lives ebbing away, without a firm purpose or sense of achievement.

In addition to the process of identity exploration, the adolescent years also mark the time where individuals begin to construe their lives in narrative terms (Bluck & Habermas, 2000). Once again, with the benefit of formal operations, adolescents have the cognitive capacity to see casual relationships among important life events and to link critical incidents across time periods into "chapters" or "phases" of their lives. This same capacity for abstraction allows them to step back from themselves and observe their own actions with a critical or reverential eye. This "observing ego" results in not only the familiar self-consciousness of adolescence but also the once-removed stance of an author observing the protagonist of an ongoing "life saga."

In one of the richer and most important contemporary theories within the field of personality, McAdams (1987, 1988, 1990, 1993, 1995, 1996, 1999, 2001) has argued that identity ultimately is the crafting of the life story across the human life span. Adolescents may begin by spinning personal fables (Elkind, 1981) that cast their lives in rather unrealistic and heroic terms, but as the events of life temper their stories, they more tentatively assemble a story that reflects frustrations along with triumphs in their lives (see also Singer, 2004b, for a discussion of the emerging body of research on narrative identity across the adult life span).

As adolescents move into young adulthood and Erikson's sixth stage of intimacy versus isolation, the life story incorporates themes of romantic relationship and efforts to establish a life partnership. Depending on each individual, the story can reflect moments of union and commitment or conflict, loneliness, and withdrawal from efforts at intimacy. In midadulthood, individuals look to the ultimate purpose or contribution of their lives, what Erikson called "generativity" in his seventh stage, and their stories increasingly take up questions of their personal legacy. This generative contribution might come in the form of child rearing but can equally be expressed through public service, aesthetic creations, and acts of commerce and industry. Here their stories can speak to the fruits of accomplishment in work and the rewards (and exhaustions) of parenting, or alternatively, the frustration of unfulfilled expectations and the stultifying routines of work or relationships that have lost their sense of meaning and purpose.

Finally, in old age, Erikson's eighth stage, individuals are prone to engage in life review, casting a backward glance that encompasses the long view of their lives. In this phase of the story, individuals ask whether the ending of their narrative brings a satisfactory closure and a sense of a job well done, a life well lived (Bornat, 2002; Butler, 1980). If older persons are unable to answer these questions in the affirmative, then they are likely to suffer from a sense of regret and despair that may cast a pall over the last phase of their lives. In contrast to stories based in the integrity of a self that retains a sense of personal control and efficacy, these despairing stories highlight the malevolent interference of others and the cruel twists of fortune that marred the possibility of a happier or more fulfilling life.

If contemporary identity is indeed this evolving and variegated life story told across the eight stages of the life cycle, what are the tools that individuals use to construct this story? Figure 4.1 identifies the four key components of McAdams's life-story theory of identity: *nuclear episodes, imagoes, ideological setting,* and *generativity script.* In addition, two fundamental dimensions underlie the other components, *thematic lines* and *narrative complexity.*

First, thematic lines are the "recurrent content clusters in stories, analogous to recurrent melodies in a complex piece of music" (McAdams,

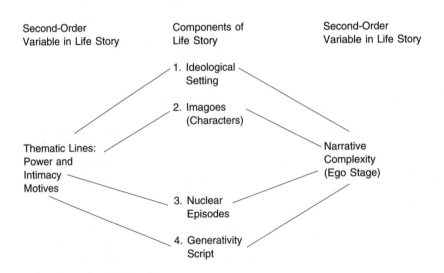

FIGURE 4.1. Life-story model of identity. From *The Remembered Self: Emotion and Memory in Personality* by Jefferson A. Singer and Peter Salovey (p. 72). Copyright 1993 by Jefferson A. Singer and Peter Salovey. Reprinted with permission of The Free Press, a Division of Simon & Schuster Adult Publishing Group. All rights reserved.

1988, p. 62). Drawing on Bakan's (1966) description of two fundamental human motives of *agency and communion,* which in turn may be traced to Freud's dictum about "love and work," McAdams has emphasized these two overarching themes of independence and relationship as dominant forces in the lives of individuals in contemporary Western societies. Many other clinical and personality psychologists have chosen to highlight the tension that emerges between these two contrasting concerns (Blatt, 1990; Fine, 1990; Hegelson & Fritz, 2000; Singer, 1988; Smelser & Erikson, 1980). *Agency* refers to the impulse in human beings to achieve independence, autonomy, and self-definition through separation. It expresses themes of competence, mastery, and power. In Chapter 3, we saw how strivings could be coded for achievement and power motives that form the core of agency. In contrast, *communion* embraces the human need for connection to others, as expressed through interdependence, affection, nurturance, helping, and sharing. The intimacy and affiliation motives discussed in Chapter 3 correspond to the essence of communion.

According to McAdams (1988), these two themes play distinct and at times conflicting roles across each individual's life course. The balance that individuals strike between the need for distinction and relationship often sets the tone for the rest of the life narrative.

The next dimension that weaves through the length of the life narrative is narrative complexity. McAdams sees complexity as reflecting the number of subplots, major and minor themes, distinctive characters, and diverse settings incorporated into the overall narrative. More complex stories also include more ambiguity, contradiction, conflict, and unresolved tension. McAdams (1988) has demonstrated that higher ego development (greater differentiation and integration of self and other) is correlated with more complex plots in life narratives.

Interwoven with narrative themes and complexity are the four life-story components. Ideological setting refers to the overall world view that guides the interpretation of events within the life story. Do individuals tend to see the world as just, people as good, and their own lives as filled with possibilities and opportunities, or do they tend toward pessimism, fearfulness, and a certain inflexibility about how life should unfold? This stance toward the world is learned early from parental models and life experiences and can often become self-fulfilling as it grows less flexible in later adulthood.

In each life story, there are recurring characters that symbolize important characteristics and roles for individuals. These *imagoes* are personal archetypes that combine different proportions of agency and communion. For example, a high-communion and low-agentic imago initially might take the form of a gentle younger sister who expresses a constant and unthreatening affection. With a sequence of similar compliant and adoring female figures emerging in an individual's narrative, one could identify this pattern as a prototypical Little Sister imago in the individual's life story.

Nuclear episodes are specific incidents that have taken their place as highly significant junctures in individuals' life stories. They can be incidents that reinforce our most critical values (e.g., a memory of a bar mitzvah or a wedding ceremony), or they can be memories of turning points and pivotal changes in individuals' lives (e.g., a memory of coming out or a memory of betrayal).

Nuclear episodes are a special category of particularly central and intense *self-defining memories*, autobiographical memories that are linked to the individual's most self-relevant and important long-term goals (Singer & Salovey, 1993). Since the collection of these memories is a key element of the Domain 3 methods used in this chapter, it is important to say a bit more about them before finishing the last aspect of McAdams's life-story theory. By discussing self-defining memories more generally, we can make better sense of where nuclear episodes fit into McAdams's model and achieve a more general understanding of the role of narrative memory in identity.

For almost two decades in my research laboratory, my colleagues and I have studied the relationship of self-defining memories to different aspects of personality. These memories are distinguished by five criteria—vividness, emotional intensity, repetition, linkage to similar memories, and their relationship to enduring concerns or unresolved conflicts. We collect these memories through the Self-Defining Memory Task (Singer & Moffitt, 1991–1992), which can be administered in either written or oral form. As we shall see, individuals are asked to imagine an intimate moment with another person in which they divulge an important experience from their past that they feel provides particular insight into who they are as a person and what is most important to them. Over multiple studies and thousands of memories (Blagov & Singer, 2004; Moffitt & Singer, 1994; Moffitt, Singer, Nelligan, Carlson, & Vyse, 1994; Singer, 1990; Singer, King, Green, & Barr, 2002; Singer & Moffitt, 1991–1992), we have been able to demonstrate reliably that this request generates memories that are highly vivid (well over 4 on a 0- to 6-point scale), emotionally powerful (scores above 4 on 0- to 6-point scales for both positive and negative emotions), and personally significant (scores approaching 5 on the 0- to 6-point scale for importance to the self). In addition, researchers have demonstrated that memories with this level of personal significance not only show linkages to clusters of other memories that share similar themes (Sutin & Robins, 2005; Thorne, Cutting, & Skaw, 1998) but also contain familiar personal scripts that can be demonstrated to emerge in individuals' other forms of narrative con-structions (e.g., in response to a request for made-up stories; Demorest & Alexander, 1992).

In mentioning the word *script*, in passing, it is worth pausing to highlight how central the concept of a script is to researchers who work in this third domain of narrative identity. If schemas, as articulated by Piaget, are organized bodies of knowledge, then scripts, as defined by both Tomkins (1979) and Schank and Abelson (1977), are schemas that contain information about sequences of events and the causal linkages that bind these sequences together. They specify rules about what precedes what in a particular type of experience, and they alert individuals to diversions from the expected sequence. For Tomkins (1979), scripts contain information, most often in an interpersonal context, about the sequence of emotions associated with a series of events. Scenes are the actual expressions of these emotion–event sequences. For example, a man may have an achievement script that follows a sequence of reaching for a goal, facing a setback, and winning ultimate success. This scripted emotional sequence of anticipation, disappointment, and joy takes the specific form of an actual scene about a high school track meet, where he started as the favorite, fell to the back of the pack, and caught the leader at the race's end.

Contemporary narrative identity researchers have studied these scripted units of personality in different forms—nuclear episodes (McAdams, 1988), memorable events (Pillemer, 1998), self-defining memories (Singer, 1995), or autobiographical memory narratives (Bluck & Gluck, 2004)—and at different levels of abstraction, ranging from the scene to the script to the life-story schema (Bluck & Habermas, 2000; Schultz, 2003). However, all of these manifestations of scripts are taken to be building blocks to narrative identity and critically related to individuals' central life goals.

For example, along with other researchers, we have reliably shown that personally important and self-defining memories are linked to individuals' goals, motives, and conflicts (Moffitt & Singer, 1994; Singer, 1990; Sutin & Robins, 2005). These findings hold for not only memories relevant to the attainment of goals we most desire, but also memories about active efforts to avoid the consequences of undesired outcomes (Moffitt & Singer, 1994).

Similarly, in examining the relationship of turning point and other significant "nuclear episode" forms of personal memories to personality, McAdams (1982; McAdams, Hoffman, Mansfield, & Day, 1996) has consistently found that individuals high in power motivation will recall turning point memories that have stronger power imagery, while individuals high in intimacy will focus more on relationship-oriented turning points. In a series of clinical case studies involving both individual and couples psychotherapy, I have demonstrated that self-defining memories are linked to central relationship themes that are expressed in both clients' intimate relationships and the transference dynamics of the therapy (Singer, 2001, 2004a; Singer & Blagov, 2004a, 2004b; Singer & Salovey, 1996; Singer & Singer, 1992, 1994). Thus, research on both self-defining memories and nuclear episodes, as one form of particularly powerful self-defining memories, has confirmed the critical role that these brief narratives of remembered experiences play in personality.

The final component of McAdams's life-story model of identity is the *generativity script*, which concerns the movement of the story toward its ultimate ending. The generativity script leads individuals to question the ultimate purpose, meaning, and significance of their lives. This questioning process often results in efforts to demonstrate that one's story has yielded a contribution or legacy that will be passed on to others.

Across the two dimensions and four components of McAdams's model is the central metaphor that identity organizes itself around the ongoing construction of this multilayered life story. Who we are is what we tell about ourselves. What we tell about ourselves is the function of our unique life history and also of the *ways of telling* we have inherited from our parents, teachers, peers, myths, mass media, national literature, religious upbringing, and other sources that define the cultural landscape we inhabit. The life story that emerges from the experiences of an upper-middle-class, college-educated professional in the United States is likely to differ in not only its specific content but also its themes, structure, and ideological settings from the life account provided by a farmer living in central Mexico. In this sense, narratives of identity take us beyond personality description (Domain 1) and dynamics (Domain 2) to the realm of meaning and the cultural context of these meaning structures. Domain 3 then, in combining Erikson's and McAdams's perspectives, is the realm of narrative identity (Singer, 2004b).

In considering Jennifer's narrative identity, how she constructs a story of her self and then attempts to extract meaning from this story, we look at both macro- and microunits of narrative. The macrounit is Jennifer's overall life story that fits within McAdams's narrative theory of identity. We examine each component of the theory from Jennifer's narrative themes all the way to her generativity script. At the same time, we look at the microunits of narratives—her self-defining memories—to determine what they might reveal about her enduring concerns or conflicts, as well as any further information we can glean from them about her emotional life, defensive organization, and capacity for meaning making. Ultimately, by combining these macro- and microanalyses, we hope to emerge with a more three-dimensional, dynamic, and living portrayal of Jennifer and her story—a portrayal that should help us take another large step toward understanding her as a person.

LIFE-STORY INTERVIEW

In order to collect information for Jennifer's life story, we employed two interview protocols that had been used in previous narrative research: the *Life-Story Questionnaires and Interviews—Appendix B* (from McAdams, 1988), and the *Identity Status Interview—Appendix B* and the *Personal History Interview—Appendix C* (from Josselson, 1996). Information on how to obtain both of these instruments is provided in Appendix A at the end of this volume. McAdams's life-story protocol consists of a series of diverse questions that encourage individuals to identify important critical incidents from their lives and to imagine these incidents as cohering into an overall narrative that comprises chapter titles, key characters, and underlying themes. These critical incidents include both "peak experiences" and "nadir experiences" that identify, respectively, the high points and low points of individuals' lives. The Life-Story Interview also includes questions that trace experiences of development through Piagetian and Eriksonian stages; that is, individuals are encouraged to recall experiences from childhood of developing competence, mastery, and autonomy, while also reflecting on evidence of trust, mentoring, and emerging peer relationships. Relative to adolescent and young adult identity formation, they are asked to contemplate the evolution of their particular religious, political, and ethic values and attitudes, as well as their increasing commitment to particular educational or vocational pursuits. At the same time that the interview takes up this identity theme, it also probes for evidence of intimacy and commitment to long-term friendships and partnerships that endure over the adult years. At many points in the interview, individuals have the opportunity to address the importance of family in their lives, both their family of origin and the families they have created or may create. Finally, the life-story protocol makes a distinct point of asking individuals to imagine their futures and to look for patterns of continuity and/or change in light of the narratives they have constructed of their lives up to the present moment.

Josselson's *Identity Status Interview* covers general areas of identity formation, including Occupation, Religion, Politics, and Sexual Values and Standards (Josselson, 1996, p. 263), and was adapted from previous interview protocols (Marcia, 1966; Schenkel & Marcia, 1972). It probes for individuals' preferences, goals, and patterns of behavior in each of these domains. The *Personal History Interview* covers the college period and adulthood, then pursues more specific questions about one's Occupational History, Education, Personal History (family, friends, romantic intimacy, child rearing), Religion, Politics, Sex, and Personal Growth. It ranges widely from questions about parents' backgrounds to current hobbies and interests.

Given the limited time my students had with their volunteer participants, I encouraged them to select a subset of questions from these protocols that would allow their participants to construct a reasonable and informative life story. Additionally, recognizing that these participants were not engaged in any kind of counseling or quasi-counseling relationship (but, alternatively, a laboratory exercise in personality research), I stressed that my student researchers needed to respect the degree of self-disclosure that participants chose to display. As a consequence, we did not obtain the same depth of information about family backgrounds and conflicts that a typical psychodynamic therapist would achieve through an extensive life-history taking. Importantly, our goal was not to collect an exhaustive amount of demographic and personal history information, but instead to sample personality from the Domain 3—Narrative Identity perspective. Accordingly, we sought to obtain a view of Jennifer as seen through the lens that she provided, as opposed to a comprehensive and "objective account" of her life. For this reason, some readers may wish for more detail about Jennifer's life and, in particular, more insight into her parents' behaviors and central concerns or themes. Yet Jennifer was highly guarded in how she talked about her family in general and her parents most of all; therefore, we are certain to disappoint readers who would like to trace her current themes back to developmental themes related to her parents' own personalities, needs, and defenses.

When we leave the laboratory assessment of personality and return to the clinical realm in Chapter 5, parent–child relationships and subsequent internalizations of representations based on these relationships occupy center stage and demonstrate what further degree of analysis is necessary to reach the fullest understanding of the whole person. In this subsequent chapter, we will need to leave Jennifer behind and return to the world of Nell, the young mother in therapy (Chapter 1). For the remainder of this chapter, though, we continue with the more circumscribed narrative that Jennifer has provided, which includes not only her life story as she conceives it but also her self-defining memories.

COLLECTING SELF-DEFINING MEMORIES

In addition to the Life-Story Interview, we asked Jennifer to recall 10 self-defining memories (Singer & Moffitt, 1991–1992; Singer & Salovey, 1993), using the latest version of the Self-Defining Memory Task (Blagov

& Singer, 2004; see Table 4.2). In previous research, we found that one needs to collect at least 5–10 self-defining memories if one hopes to discern reliable patterns of content, theme, and structure across the group of memories. Normally, after individuals recall their 10 self-defining memories, they rate the memories for their current emotional responses on 12 emotion adjectives and also indicate the vividness and importance of the memories. For the purposes of this individual assessment, we simply asked Jennifer to rate each memory from 0 to 2 for how positively and from 0 to 2 for how negatively she felt in recalling it today. We also had her consider all 10 memories as a whole and rank them from 1 to 10 for their importance to her. Jennifer wrote each of her 10 memories on a separate sheet of paper and placed her emotion ratings and ranking at the bottom of each sheet.

TABLE 4.2. Self-Defining Memory Task

This task concerns the recall of a special kind of personal memory called a self-defining memory, which has the following attributes:

1. It is at least 1 year old.
2. It is a memory from your life that you remembered very clearly and that still feels important to you even as you think about it.
3. It is a memory about an important enduring theme, issue, or conflict from your life. It is a memory that helps explain who you are as an individual and might be the memory you would tell someone else if you wanted that person to understand you in a profound way.
4. It is a memory linked to other similar memories that share the same theme or concern.
5. It may be a memory that is positive or negative, or both, in how it makes you feel. The only important aspect is that it leads to strong feelings.
6. It is a memory that you have thought about many times. It should be familiar to you like a picture you have studied or a song (happy or sad) you have learned by heart.

To understand best what a self-defining memory is, imagine that you have just met someone you like very much and you are going for a walk together. Each of you is very committed to helping the other get to know the "real you." You are not trying to play a role or to strike a pose. While, inevitably, we say things that present a picture of ourselves that might not be completely accurate, imagine that you are making every effort to be honest. In the course of the conversation, you describe a memory that you feel conveys powerfully how you have come to be the person you currently are. It is precisely this memory, which you tell the other person and simultaneously repeat to yourself, that constitutes a self-defining memory.

On the following pages, you will be asked to recall and write 10 self-defining memories.

The combination of the Life-Story Interview and the Self-defining Memory Task took 2 hours to complete.

ANALYSIS OF THE LIFE STORY

There is an extraordinary range of analyses that one might bring to the narrative data generated by the life-story and personal history protocols, as well as by the Self-Defining Memory Task. As McAdams (1988, 2001) has detailed, the incidents described in the Life-Story Interview can be coded for themes of achievement, power, intimacy and affiliation, along with other social motives. The protocols can also be coded for narrative complexity, which is correlated with ego development (McAdams, 1988). One can identify Redemption and Contamination scripts and significant imagoes (McAdams, Reynolds, Lewis, Patten, & Bowman, 2001). For the Identity Status and Personal History Interviews, as Josselson (1996) demonstrates, identity status, as well as other significant agentic and communal themes, can be determined. As my colleagues and I have detailed (Blagov & Singer, 2004; Singer & Blagov, 2002; Singer & Moffitt, 1991–1992), self-defining memories can be coded for the specificity of their narrative structure, their content (see Thorne & McLean, 2001), their integrative meaning, and their emotion. All of these coding systems are available through the published literature or in coding manuals available from the authors cited. For excellent overviews of how to perform content analysis and the coding of narrative material, I would recommend three valuable sources—Alexander (1990), Smith (2000), and Josselson, Lieblich, and McAdams (2003). Each of these volumes provides specific guidelines and tools that allow one to draw from a menu of quantitative and qualitative techniques for content analysis of narratives.

In my personality seminar, I urged students to use McAdams's life-story model of identity as the starting point for examining the life-history protocols. In other words, one should look to define the overall story (the beginning and ending point at the present time) that the participants have imposed on their life-history information. After defining this narrative and its "chapters," one could look for the underlying presence of agency versus communion themes by more careful examination of the critical incidents that comprise the life narrative. These incidents might share common sequences of actions–outcomes–emotions that define prototypical scripts for individuals. One could also look for repetitive characterizations or archetypal figures that lead to the identification of participants' imagoes. Finally, with regard to narrative complexity, one could evaluate the overall narrative for its degree of ambiguity, nuance, divergence, and relative simplicity. Though all of these life-story variables can be evaluated in a quantitative and nomothetic fashion (e.g., McAdams & de St. Aubin, 1992), our current goal was to look more idiographically and descriptively at their relative significance in Jennifer's life story.

Yet before engaging in these various analyses, we need to recall and elaborate the basic setting of Jennifer's life—the demographic details that locate her in the most rooted of ways in a particular time and place. It is time to return to the Jennifer who exists beyond the inventories, striving lists, and rating scales that have allowed us to construct her image thus far (but please recall that critical details of her story have been changed to protect her anonymity). Perhaps the place to start is to describe the circumstances of her initial assessment session and whatever external impressions emerged.

Due to feeling under the weather from a cold, Jennifer asked the student examiner to meet for the session in her dormitory room. The examiner reported that her room was filled with brightly colored posters of cartoon characters (e.g., Tweety Bird and Mickey Mouse), as well as assorted stuffed animals. Given Jennifer's tendency to present herself to the examiner in a rather serious and reserved light, the "little girl" quality of the room was a bit surprising. The other salient initial impression, which I also mentioned in Chapter 2, this volume, is Jennifer's unusual physical beauty. Her long, straight, dark hair, olive complexion, high cheekbones, and the regularity of her features, as well as her height, slender frame, and athleticism, could easily type her for an actress or model.

Jennifer traced her heritage to a mix of Irish and French Canadian background. Her father, the oldest son from a closely knit Irish Catholic family, runs a highly successful real estate business in their New England community. His original family came to this country in the late 19th century but has lived successfully in this same town now over several generations. Her mother does not work outside the home at present, but she is heavily involved in taking care of her own father, who lives in a nearby assisted-living complex. Interestingly, Jennifer's grandfather has a history of anxiety; she did not specify whether her mother shares this same vulnerability as well. Her mother also helps her father with his business at times. Jennifer has one brother, a year older, who is a senior at her same college. Due to a year of travel between high school and college, he is now in the same year that she is. At the time of the interview, both Jennifer and her brother were members of their college soccer teams, and each has a strong record of athletic accomplishment.

Jennifer described her family as very close, and many of her father's siblings, their spouses, and children live near to their home. She described her parents as "doing everything just right." They were caring, never pressured her, and always did whatever they could do to boost her self-esteem. Though their home is a few hours away from the college, Jennifer reported that she still sees her parents one or two times a week. In fact, her parents' record of virtually never missing her or her brother's athletic events dates all the way back to elementary school. They even attend their out-of-town college games.

Having laid a basic groundwork for Jennifer's life story, we can turn to one of the key questions from both McAdams's protocol and Josselson's Personal History Interview—a request for participants to describe their lives in a series of thematic chapters. Table 4.3 presents Jennifer's Life-Story Chapters and Theme. From Jennifer's "Table of Contents," we see a fairly typical progression from childhood behavior to a latency period focus on athletic accomplishment and academics, leading up to her first college experience. The final two chapters suggest some significant variations from the typical trajectory of the upper-middle-class college-student narrative. First, Jennifer made a decision to transfer, which though not markedly unusual, does suggest a sufficient level of dissatisfaction to warrant attention. Second, her final chapter stresses family rather than themes that might reflect a normative increase in autonomy and independence (e.g., applying to graduate school, interviewing for jobs, travel, moving to a city). Yet depending on sociocultural mores, one might attribute this last chapter title to an ethnic and cultural emphasis on family unity as opposed to a sign of difficulty. This last point receives some support from Jennifer's life-story theme of "family and its importance in life."

We can already see how a Domain 3 analysis sheds new light on some our previous hypotheses about Jennifer. The particular Domain 1 and Domain 2 measures that we selected do not necessarily tap into information about ethnic or cultural influences and traditions. In the de facto context of an upper-middle-class Anglo American culture, where

---

TABLE 4.3. Jennifer's Life-Story Chapters and Theme

Chapter 1—Hyperactive Child

Chapter 2—Performing

Chapter 3—Figure Skating

Chapter 4—High School

Chapter 5—First College Experience

Chapter 6—Transferring

Chapter 7—Family

Overall theme—Family and Its Importance in Life

---

independence is the coin of the realm in Northeastern liberal arts college environments, Jennifer's very high Agreeableness and low Conscientiousness, combined with her lack of agentic strivings and her emphasis on family and familiar routines, make her seem like someone stuck in the identity formation process, possibly mired in a state of diffusion or foreclosure (Marcia, 1966; Waterman, 1982). Yet the ethnic tradition of her close-knit Irish Catholic family places loyalty and involvement with family at a premium. Given her parents' devotion to her (e.g., traveling all over the Northeast to attend her sporting events), it is not surprising that she might see her next move after college to be a return to her family home. Without this Domain 3 context of how she understands her own sense of identity in relation to her family and its cultural values, we might place too much emphasis on the more general information provided at the Traits and Characteristic Adaptations domains. Acknowledging this point does not dismiss the clear difficulties that Jennifer has with social anxiety and envisioning a future for herself, but it does temper one's rush to emphasize her reluctance to separate from her family and strike out on an independent course.

Let us learn more about how Jennifer filled in the details of each chapter of her life. In Chapter 1—Hyperactive Child, she recalled her uninhibited, "goofy" behavior that would annoy her older brother. In those days, she saw herself as the opposite of her more serious and obedient brother. By the time that she entered grade school (Chapter 2—Performing), ice-skating, dancing, and soccer dominated her life. She recalled that period as a time in which she had many friends and was often a leader of her peer group. As she advanced through middle school and junior high, her world had become organized around competitive figure-skating, though she still managed to play in soccer leagues as well. She devoted herself to daily practice regimens and remembered how she raced from one athletic event to the next. The nature of her sporting experiences changed from performing for fun to a much more pressurized and competitive climate. She still recalled having a good circle of friends but admitted that she had little time to share with them given her rigorous training.

Chapter 4—High School marked a major transition in Jennifer's life. First, two very large regional middle schools merged to create an even larger high school. She found the size of the building and the numbers of fellow students overwhelming. Second, she started to experience herself as shy and less outgoing. Though she met many new people and made new friends, she resented the familiar high school emphases on cliques and popularity. Many people seemed to respond to her in a superficial way, seeking to befriend or, in the case of males, date her, but she felt that they did not take the time to learn who she really was. She not only continued to devote time to figure-skating but also began to balance these efforts with involvement on the high school soccer team. Increasingly, she found herself more comfortable with a team sport rather than being the single focus of attention that figure-skating required.

It was during early high school (age 14–15) that Jennifer first detected a shift in her self-esteem and general satisfaction with herself. In contrast to the confident, outgoing child she had once been, she started to experience a great deal of self-doubt and even self-loathing. She feared others' disapproval and criticism. In particular, she grew to hate her appearance and would often hide in her room and cry about her self-perceived ugliness. Her anxiety and insecurity were powerful enough that her parents brought her to a therapist. She received diagnoses of an anxiety disorder and a body dysmorphic disorder, indicating a highly distorted image of her own appearance (Phillips, 2001). Jennifer explained that she still cannot bear to look in a mirror, and she avoids having her picture taken at all costs. During these years, she first started to have fits of sobbing if confronted by an image of herself in a bathroom mirror. Her close friends soon learned to distract her if she came anywhere near a mirror. When out at a restaurant or other public venue, they would always go with her to the bathroom to prevent her catching a glimpse of her reflection and breaking down.

With this extreme concern about her appearance, Jennifer was clearly at risk for an eating disorder, yet she did not mention this specific problem in detailing her history. It may be that her decision to concentrate on a high-contact team sport steered her away from the eating difficulties that are not uncommon for individual-sport female athletes (e.g., gymnasts, dancers, cross-country runners). On the other hand, it may that she chose not to disclose this aspect of her history due to the shame that accompanies this behavior.

In an effort to address her bouts of sobbing and anxiety, she had tried and discontinued several different kinds of antidepressants over the years. She felt that none of them had been particularly effective in lifting her mood or helping her manage her anxiety. Though she has had little success with medication, she indicated that her depression had been building in recent months and that she might request another course of treatment soon.

Given the emotional struggles that emerged in high school, it is not surprising that the Chapter 5—First College Experience did little to settle Jennifer's anxieties. Leaving her family behind was difficult enough, but the social environment of the university she had chosen also posed some problems for her. Since the university had once had a strong religious affiliation, it still restricted the students to single-sex dormitories, which she felt inhibited informal contact among the male and female students. All socializing was based around large mixers that placed an emphasis on appearance and casual encounters. Despite the distance, she found that she was driving home almost every weekend. She made a few friendships, but none of the depth that she had experienced with her hometown friends. Her focus soon turned to demonstrating her academic strength in order to transfer to her brother's college.

Her academic success led to Chapter 6—Transferring and a period of initial nervousness, followed by much greater happiness at her new school. She tried out for and made the soccer team, which allowed her to make a new set of very positive women friends. The college was smaller and closer to her home, not to mention allowing her nearly daily contact with her brother. Jennifer found the academic work more challenging and needed to work even harder, but she also learned to accept that grades in the B to B+ range represented a good result for her. Overall, in both academic and social areas, she felt that she had made an excellent decision to transfer and was proud of her ability to take constructive action in her life.

The last phase, Chapter 7—Family, emphasized Jennifer's ongoing relationship with her parents and extended family in her home community, and her intention to move back there after graduation. She plans to work once she returns home but has no clear image of what immediate work she might find.

As part of the Life-Story Interview, Jennifer was asked to indicate what the overarching theme and the overall philosophy of her life story might be. She responded by saying that the central theme was her family, and maintaining the comfortable atmosphere that her family had created. She added that her philosophy is "to be how you are comfortable; don't cater to how others want you to be." As an example, she pointed out that she goes home frequently (often once a week) because it makes her happy, and she does not care what others say about this choice. In an almost defiant fashion, which was unusual for her in the interview, she stated that her going home "doesn't prove anything."

Additional questioning revealed some further aspects of Jennifer's life history that supplement the rather bare narrative that she constructed. Regarding her family, Jennifer described a particular mentally disabled cousin who lives with one of her aunts. Jennifer is very close to this cousin and has volunteered in Special Olympics events to help her. She describes this cousin as always good-natured and full of love for all aspects of life. It is indeed possible that Jennifer's strong commitment to strivings about open-mindedness and not judging others is connected to her experiences with this cousin.

Jennifer also indicated that though she is very close to both parents, she has always felt a special bond with her father. She described him as sharing the same "goofy" sense of humor that she first mentioned in her chapter on childhood. Her father has been a strong source of support and the prime cheerleader in all her endeavors. She sees no connection whatsoever between her insecurity and the wellspring of positive recognition he has provided. In general, she mentioned that she strongly identifies with the humor and values of her father's whole side of the family.

Another previously omitted topic was a discussion of the role of romantic relationships in her life. It turns out that despite her striking appearance and her ability to have ongoing close friendships, Jennifer had never actually dated in either high school or college. She explained that this lack of relationships was not due to any kind of pressure or social prohibitions set by her family, or by religious strictures. She traced the explanation to her anxiety and her need to have powerful control over the impressions that she would make in any dating situation.

As we probed her future a bit more, it emerged that Jennifer's parents wish that she had a more definite plan and hope that she will soon take some concrete steps toward defining a future career or educational goal. When pushed about where she sees herself in 5–10 years, Jennifer could not articulate a specific image, but she did mention a possibility that she would move to Florida to escape the cold winters of the Northeast. However, she admitted that the distance from her family made such a move unlikely. She did anticipate that she would get married and have children. She envisioned herself working part-time, while she raised her children. Regarding the kind of work she might do, Jennifer could imagine herself working with young children or with elderly and/or disabled people in some social service capacity.

Since my request for self-defining memories evoked memories that overlapped with a number of the critical events that Jennifer recalled for her life-story narrative, it makes sense to discuss the memories first and then provide an overall analysis of Jennifer through the lens of McAdams's (1988) life-story theory of identity.

SELF-DEFINING MEMORIES

Memory Specificity

Similar to her life story, Jennifer's self-defining memories are striking for their relative sparseness of detail and overall brevity (see Table 4.4 for her 10 self-defining memories ranked in order of importance). Applying the scoring methods outlined in the Self-Defining Memory coding manual (Singer & Blagov, 2002; see Appendix A), we might begin by coding the 10 memories for the degree of narrative specificity.

TABLE 4.4. Jennifer's Self-Defining Memories

1. Finding out that my grandfather had died. This happened during my freshman year in college. It was the first time that I had lost a family member. (Positive—0/Negative—2)

2. Transferring to a new college. The school that I had previously attended and my current school are extremely different, so it was a change of lifestyle. Socially, it was a big adjustment. (Positive—2/Negative—0)

3. Deciding to join a highly competitive figure-skating club. It was a huge commitment and one that changed my adolescent years. (Left out emotion ratings)

4. Going on our first family vacation with my father's side of the family. This was the first time that I had been together with all 20 of my relatives for an entire week. It brought my family closer together. (Positive—2/Negative—0)

5. Beginning to feel negatively about myself. As a child, I had much self-confidence, but as I entered my teenage years, that confidence faded and I became insecure. This made life more difficult because it is something that affects me on a daily basis. (Positive—0/Negative—2)

6. Going on vacation to Florida with my mother for the first time. This was the first time that my mother and I had been alone together for an extended period of time. (Positive—2/Negative—0)

7. Being dropped off at college my freshman year. I had never been away from my family before, and I knew that I would not be able to see them as often as I would like. This was the first time that I had to be completely independent, and I did not know anyone at college. (Positive—1/Negative—1)

8. Climbing into my brother's crib after my parents put us to bed. We would then fall asleep in the crib together. (Positive—2/Negative—0)

9. Deciding to play soccer after I transferred. I knew it would be a much higher level than I had played at. I decided to challenge myself and play. (Positive—2/Negative—1)

10. Graduating high school and having to leave the friends I had grown up with. I had to leave a situation that I was comfortable in for one that was uncertain (college). (Positive—1/Negative—1)

Note. Each memory was ranked by Jennifer for how positively (0–2) and how negatively (0–2) it made her feel while currently recalling it.

Narrative specificity captures the degree to which a particular self-defining memory makes reference to a unique occurrence located in a particular moment of time and traceable to a specific location. The event is typically brief in duration, containing happenings of less than a day or a night and the following morning. The overall event is recounted with an uninterrupted unity as a bounded incident.

In contrast, nonspecific memory narratives can take two primary forms—*episodic* and *generic*. The *episodic* memory narrative usually spans more than a day and often much longer: a weeklong holiday, a summer's vacation, a junior year abroad, a period of unemployment. Actions and events are generalized within this time frame and often lack the imagery and detail of the specific memory. For example, the following is an episodic memory:

> "When I was in second grade, Mom had to go to the hospital for 2 months, because she had my brother Todd prematurely. I had to help Dad by helping clean, cook, do laundry, and take care of my brother Jim. Although I was only helping my dad, it was still a lot of responsibility to help with the house."

The *generic* memory is composed of equivalent events that are repeated over time intervals that extend beyond a year's time. These repeated events fuse together, blending the same characters, settings, happenings, and emotions. The following is an example of a generic memory:

> "I remember, when I was little, going to pick pumpkins with my mother. Every Halloween, we would drive a long way to a friend's farm. I loved searching around with my mom to try and find the perfect pumpkin. It never really mattered how good they were the next day, but it was the fun we had searching for them that I appreciate."

As we shall see, applying this coding system to Jennifer's 10 self-defining memories is extremely simple and strikingly informative. Looking at her 10 memories, it is clear that she has chosen an episodic narrative structure for all of her memories. This is highly unusual; in previous research on thousands of self-defining memories, we have documented that 80–85% of the memories recalled will be rated as specific and that individuals asked to recall 10 memories will seldom have more than two or three nonspecific memories (Blagov & Singer, 2004; Moffitt & Singer, 1994; Singer & Moffitt, 1991–1992). In Jennifer's case, she has only two memories that might even possibly be tied to a specific moment in time ("finding out my grandfather died" and "being dropped off at college my freshman year"), yet in both cases, no additional imagery or specific details are provided that allow one to classify these as unique, specific memories. Given the more general description that follows the mention of these events, it is not at all clear whether Jennifer is referring to the days or months that followed these pivotal events in her life or to a specific memory of these events that includes imagery of a moment or moments in time. Due to this lack of specificity, each of these memories is scored as a nonspecific episodic memory, and both contribute to her high nonspecific memory total. In our efforts to understand Jennifer, we might then ask: What does it mean that she has provided only episodic memories and no specific self-defining memories?

Over the years, my colleagues and I have studied the relationship of self-defining memory specificity to individual differences in personality. One possibility is that depressed individuals might have a pervasive difficulty in recalling specific memories. The British psychologist Mark Williams has repeatedly documented the problem of overgeneral recall in suicidal and chronically depressed individuals (Moore, Watts, & Williams, 1988; Williams, 1996, 2004; Williams & Broadbent, 1986; Williams & Dritschel, 1988; Williams & Scott, 1988). He has suggested that this memory specificity deficit might be due to an overlearned strategy adopted by individuals who have been exposed to extensive negative events or powerful traumatic situations in order to preempt the retrieval of painful experiences. Although it was first applied to negative material, over time, it generalized as threat-protective device activated by retrieval of any specific information. Alternatively, one might suggest an "effort" explanation, in that individuals who are acutely depressed may not be able to exert the cognitive effort to retrieve a specific memory; they simply stop their search process at more general levels of memory recall. This argument seems plausible, but Williams has been able to find the memory deficit in chronically depressed individuals who are no longer in an acute state of depression (Williams, 1996).

In applying Williams's work on depression and overgeneral memory to self-defining memories, we looked at the possibility that a lack of specificity in self-defining memories might be associated with a tendency toward dysphoric mood (Moffitt et al., 1994). Using a within-participants design, we asked mildly depressed and nondepressed individuals to recall two memories, one positive and the other negative, and then looked at the degree of specificity in each memory. We found that the mildly depressed individuals were less likely to recall a positive specific memory than the nondepressed individuals but did not differ in their number of negative specific memories. Although this finding differs from some of Williams's previous findings and predictions, it does fit well with a line of research on mood and memory (Blaney, 1986; Rusting, 1998; Singer & Salovey, 1988) that suggests nondepressed individuals repair their negative moods by recalling positive memories. The Moffitt et al. (1994) study pointed to one reason why depressed individuals might have difficulty with this mood repair process; the positive memories they recall are less vivid and evocative than the specific negative memories they can recall. Josephson, Singer, and Salovey (1996) provided additional confirmation for this mood repair by memory hypothesis, although, in this study, we did not examine memory specificity. We induced a negative mood in nondepressed and depressed individuals by showing them a film clip of the saddest scenes from the film *Terms of Endearment*, then asking each participant to recall two memories. Nondepressed individuals were much more likely than depressed individuals to recall a negative memory followed by a mood-repairing positive memory; in contrast, the depressed individuals were more likely to recall two negative memories consecutively. One possibility, then, for Jennifer's high number of nonspecific memories could be her tendency toward depression and her current sense that she is moving back into a more acute depression. Yet if that were the case, it is not clear whether we might have expected her to have fewer specific positive memories, as the Moffitt et al. (1994) study suggests, or fewer specific memories in general, as Williams's theory predicts.

An alternative possibility hinted at by Williams's theory about an overlearned general style is that individuals who are defended against negative emotion or the expression of strong emotion of any kind might have fewer specific memories. Recently, Blagov and Singer (2004) examined the relationship of memory specificity to this defensive personality style, which I discussed earlier as repressive defensiveness (see Chapter 3, section on the Weinberger Adjustment Inventory—Short Form [WAI-SF] and its Repressive Defensiveness scale). Weinberger (1998) defined *Repressive Defensiveness* as a tendency to deny any deviation from social expectations and an unwillingness to acknowledge the existence of negative outcomes in one's life. There is some previous evidence (Davis & Schwartz, 1987) that individuals high in repression recall fewer emotional memories and limit themselves to memories from more recent periods in their lives. Singer and Salovey (1993) also reported some preliminary data that pointed to less specific recall in individuals with a repressive style.

In the Blagov and Singer (2004) study, 104 participants recalled 10 self-defining memories and also filled out the WAIS-SF. Using our specificity coding system, the number of specific memories for each person was correlated with his or her Repressive Defensiveness score. There was a significant negative correlation, indicating that a higher degree of Repressive Defensiveness was associated with more nonspecific memories. Interestingly, the emotional quality of the memories, as rated by the participants, was not linked to their level of defensiveness.

The combination of these findings suggests that repressive defensiveness may reflect more how individuals structure their memory narratives and less what they choose to remember or claim to feel about the memory. Perhaps the initial repressive concern is to preempt "looking" at specific events altogether (by clinging to a nonspecific structure).

Events that make it through this filter have been "sanitized" of vivid and self-threatening imagery, regardless of the putative emotion associated with them. In other words, individuals can recall the content in general terms and even assign a negative emotion to them but ultimately do not "reexperience" or fully engage with the memory.

Jennifer's Repressive Defensiveness score in Chapter 3 was in the 95th percentile for her age group. This extreme Repressive Defensiveness score fits the Blagov and Singer (2004) findings remarkably well, since she generated no specific memories. The evidence from this Domain 3 narrative analysis strongly supports the converging picture of Jennifer as someone who is reluctant to acknowledge any conduct or emotional experience in her life that might engender disapproval or criticism.

Memory Meaning

Having examined Jennifer's memories for their narrative structure, we may next consider what we have defined as *integrative meaning* (Blagov & Singer, 2004; Singer & Blagov, 2002), which refers to individuals' tendency to step back from their recollections and assign a lesson, moral, or interpretation to the remembered experience. Anyone can recall a memory, but taking the step to attach a meaning to a memory is a separate cognitive process. Theorists (e.g., Robinson, 1986) have suggested that the creation of meaning from memory helps to regulate moods and assists communication in intimate relationships. Making meaning of past struggles and sharing this insight has been found to predict positive self-regard in college students (Debats, Drost, & Hansen, 1995), less grief over time in bereaved spouses (Bauer & Bonanno, 2001), and well-being, a sense of growth, and enhanced ego development in parents of disabled children (King, Scollon, Ramsey, & May, 2000).

In agreement with Pillemer (1998) and the work of Thorne, McLean, and Lawrence (2004), Singer and Blagov (2002) developed the more general construct of *integrative memories*: narratives in which individuals take the additional step of ascribing meaning to their memories by relating them to lessons about the self, important relationships, or life in general. We have proposed (Singer & Blagov, 2004a, 2004b) that the meaning-making process in the construction of self-defining memories enables memory to affect the self through the linkage of memory to important self-relevant goals (also see Conway & Pleydell-Pearce, 2000; Conway, Singer, & Tagini, 2004).

The Singer and Blagov (2002) coding manual allows one to code the integrative meanings in memories reliably, which then offers the researcher the opportunity to correlate the number of integrative memories generated by an individual with other measures of personality. Table 4.5 provides examples of the two types of self-defining memories: integrative and nonintegrative.

Looking at Jennifer's self-defining memories, we can code each memory for the presence or absence of integrative meanings. On first look, it might seem that Jennifer has included some integrative statements or lesson learning in her memory narratives. If we examine memories 3, 4, and 5 in Table 4.4, we read language that almost seems integrative:

3. " . . . It was a huge commitment and one that changed my adolescent years."
4. " . . . It brought my family closer together."
5. " . . . This made life more difficult, because it is something that affects me on a daily basis."

Yet when we consider these statements more carefully, we see that no life lesson, moral, or identifiable meaning emerges from these statements. We know that memory 3 changed her adolescent years, but not in what way. In memory 4, we see that the events brought

TABLE 4.5. Examples of Integrative versus Nonintegrative
Self-Defining Memories

Integrative memory

When I was 14, my friend and I were caught smoking pot in the school lavatory. We were suspended from school and almost arrested. The worst part of the memory was the night I had to sit down and talk about what I had done with my father. I still can see the pain and confusion in his face, more those feelings than anger. The big thing was that I had told him that I never used pot and here the truth had come out. It was like all the years of trust that we had had were gone in one day or least that was how it felt at the time. I remember I made a vow that night that even if I did something against his wishes, I would not lie about it. I really learned that night that trust with people you love is even more important than trying to look good or seeming perfect in their eyes. Ever since then, I have tried to be a more honest person.

Nonintegrative memory

I remember when my grandfather passed away. It was one of the saddest days of my life. I remember my mother standing by the telephone and crying, while my father rubbed her back. My little brother came over and hugged my leg, while I tried not to sniffle too. The next few days were a blur of family members crying and hugging, the funeral, and people dropping by. It seemed like it rained every day and I felt like I could never quite get warm.

her family closer together, but there is no additional lesson or abstracted meaning to draw from this statement. Jennifer's acknowledgment in memory 5 that her insecurity affects her on a daily basis does not lead her to state a conclusion or inference derived from this observation. Aside from these memories, the other seven memories simply acknowledge "firsts" in her life, "transitions," or "decisions," with no effort to reflect at a higher level of abstraction on what these events have taught her about herself or life in general. For these reasons, Jennifer would receive a score of 0/10 for the number of integrative memories she produced. Similar to her score for memory specificity, Jennifer's results are unusual compared to those of a sample of college student peers. In a similar study of life lessons and insights attached to self-defining memories, Thorne et al. (2004) found that approximately 20–25% of the self-defining memories they collected had meaning statements attached to them. Our own research (Blagov & Singer, 2004) found that between 20 and 40% of self-defining memories are likely to be integrative. What then might Jennifer's striking absence of integrative memories mean?

Previous researchers have found that the capacity to learn from memory and to incorporate life lessons into ongoing self-knowledge are characteristics associated with individuals rated by others as "wise" and "well-adjusted" (Staudinger, 2001; Staudinger, Lopez, & Baltes, 1997). This kind of ruminative insight is certainly one of the prized goals of any psychotherapy, whether insight-oriented or cognitive-behavioral. In broad terms, then, the ability to generate integrative meanings from narrative memory should be associated with higher levels of socioemotional maturity and personal adjustment.

Drawing once more on the WAI-SF, we might return to Weinberger's (1998) formulation of moderate self-restraint as reflective of optimal personal adjustment. Recalling his framework from Chapter 3, we find that individuals with high levels of self-restraint are likely to be overcontrolled and too rigid with regard to their expression of emotion and impulses, while individuals with low levels of self-restraint would be likely to be undercontrolled, impulsive, and more prone to emotional outbursts and acting-out behavior. Moderate levels of self-restraint allow for flexibility of response to social demands and an ability to modulate open expression of feelings, with concern for the effect of emotional displays and behaviors on others. Based on this model, we hypothesized that individuals with higher numbers of integrative memories should score in the moderate range on Weinberger's WAI-SF Self-Restraint scale, while individuals with very high or very low scores in Self-Restraint would display few integrative memories. As Figure 4.2 displays,

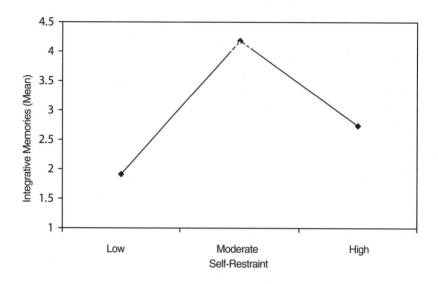

FIGURE 4.2. Relationship of integrative memories to self-restraint. Adapted from Blagov and Singer (2004). Copyright 2004 by Blackwell. Adapted by permission.

this is exactly what we found across our sample of 104 participants (Blagov & Singer, 2004).

Applying these findings to Jennifer's protocol, we see again an accurate match between the previous research and her specific case. Jennifer scored in the 80–90% range on Self-Restraint, locating her in the extremely overcontrolled range. As discussed in Chapter 3, this result suggests that Jennifer's proneness to conformity and an externalizing defensive style does not allow her to profit from the potential lessons that her memories might teach her.

Memory Emotion

Another feature of the Self-Defining Memory Task is that individuals rate their current emotional response to each memory they recall. Looking at Jennifer's emotional responses (measured on separate 3-point scales of positive and negative emotion), we can see that, overall, she rated four memories as purely positive, two as purely negative, and three as a mixture of positive and negative. She neglected to provide ratings for her memory about joining a competitive figure-skating club. Three of her four positive memories make reference to positive experiences with her immediate family and/or relatives (the Florida vacation with her mother; the cruise with her father's side of family; climbing into her brother's crib); the other positive memory concerned her transfer to her new college. This is a hopeful sign given that it is a recent memory that reinforces the value of her taking action to change a negative situation. Her two purely negative memories concern the loss of her grandfather and the beginning of her negative perception of herself. All three mixed-emotions memories involve acts of self-assertion—graduating high school; being dropped off for college; and deciding to play soccer at her new college. Interestingly, these three memories rank in the bottom four of Jennifer's memories relative to importance.

Personality and clinical researchers have consistently examined the relationship of emotional responses to memories and individuals' proneness to depression (Blaney, 1986; Matt, Vazquez, & Campbell, 1992; Rusting, 1998; Singer & Salovey, 1988). In our recent work (Blagov & Singer, 2004), we found that individuals who scored higher in Self-Reported Distress on the WAI-SF recalled memories associated with higher levels of negative emotion and lower levels of positive emotion (for similar connections between emotional dispositions and memory emotional tone, see Sutin & Robins, 2005). Additionally, individuals who reported higher distress had more memories about disrupted relationships and loss, as well as threat of physical injury and illness. They also reported fewer memories about successful achievement in their lives. Considering that the majority of Jennifer's memories are mixed or negative (5) versus strongly positive (4), and that most individuals tend to show a strong differential in the reverse, her memory–emotion profile does indeed seem congruent with that of an individual who is showing depressive tendencies.

Memory Content

The final dimension of self-defining memories—memory content—is the one most squarely linked to questions of identity and narrative in context. Looking at memory content brings us back to the overall life-story narrative collected in the life story interview and therefore links the memory and life-story components of Domain 3. There are three major ways we can study the content of Jennifer's 10 self-defining memories: (1) we can simply group memories into content categories based on a content coding system for self-defining memories developed by Thorne and McLean (2001; for information on how to obtain this system, see Appendix A); (2) we can code the memories for agentic and communal themes through a memory thematic coding system available from McAdams (2002; see Table 4.6); and (3) we can apply a more interpretive and less systematic effort to identify Tomkins-like "scripts" within the memories.

TABLE 4.6. Excerpts from McAdams's (2002) Manual for Coding
Autobiographical Episodes for Themes of Agency and Communion

Agency

1. Achievement/Responsibility (AR). The protagonist in the story expresses
significant success in achievement tasks or assumes important responsibilities. He
or she displays feelings of pride, confidence, and mastery. These major successes
are usually in achievement settings, such as school or work. The protagonist is
striving to meet a high standard of excellence.

Examples of AR

• A student works hard to perfect a short story for a class assignment. He spends
  hours polishing word choice, getting the imagery right, and so on.
• An executive meets his annual goals for the company.
• A young boy builds a tree house, and he is very proud of his accomplishment.
• A student masters a class on computer programming.

2. Power/Impact (PI). The protagonist asserts his or her impact and/or influence
on others. This impact is manifest in various vivid forms including aggression,
argument, persuasion, control, and impression making. Through expressing his or
her will and having an impact on others or the environment, the protagonist feels
powerful and masterful. The effect may be positive or negative. Often PI themes
are associated with efforts at leadership or the protagonist's ability to mobilize
others to pursue his or her interests.

Examples of PI

• A politician pushes through a piece of legislation.
• A woman persuades her friends to change their views about a controversial
  topic.
• A bully beats up other children on the playground.
• Somebody saves somebody else's life.

3. Self-Insight (SI). The protagonist achieves an important insight or moment of
self-understanding through the event. As a result, the protagonist expresses a
growth in maturity, wisdom, or self-actualization. This insight leads to a
commitment to a new set of ideals, goals, or plans that moves the individual in a
new and more positive direction.

Examples of SI

• A woman comes to see her life's mission as being an artist. She quits her job,
  sets up a studio, and strives to actualize her dream.
• A young man experiences a religious conversion that provides him with new
  insight into his own life.
• A middle-aged man realizes that he is being exploited by his current employer.
  He breaks away from the firm and embarks upon a new line of work, more in
  keeping with his life goals.
• A woman comes to the conclusion that she has wasted 20 years of her life in a
  desperate drive for material well-being. She decides to dedicate her life to
  helping others.

TABLE 4.6. (*continued*)

4. Status/Victory (SV). The protagonist attains a heightened status or prestige in relation to others. This status always involves a "winning" against peer competitors. It can be in any form of contest—academic, athletic, performing arts, and so on. Achieving success or doing well is not sufficient for this category. The status change must be described as a victory or triumph in relationship to others.

Examples of SV

- A young woman is elected homecoming queen.
- An actor wins a coveted lead part in an upcoming play.
- A student graduates from college with special honors (e.g., *magna cum laude*).
- The quarterback completes a crucial pass, which gives his team the victory in the football game.

Communion

5. Love/Friendship (LF). A protagonist experiences an episode that involves an increase in love or friendship toward another person. A relationship between people grows in intimacy.

Examples of LF

- Two friends feel that they grow emotionally closer to each other after spending time together on a vacation.
- A man proposes to a woman (or vice versa).
- A woman describes her marriage to a wonderful man as the high point of her life.
- A man marvels at the love and commitment his wife has given him over the past 40 years.

6. Dialogue (DG). A character in the story undergoes a reciprocal and noninstrumental form of communication or dialogue with another person or group of others. This dialogue is most often a conversation between people. The conversation must be in the interest of genuine exchange, as opposed to an instrumental reason (e.g., scheduling a meeting, conducting a transaction, replying to a survey). Conversations for helping others (e.g., advice, counseling, mentoring) do count for this category.

Examples of DG

- We sat across from each other and tossed ideas back and forth, ideas of what we thought the plays were about.
- Sara and I had been writing letters to each other all summer.
- We drank a carafe of wine and had a memorable conversation about love and parents.
- My peak experience was both a time of sadness and joy. Sadness because my friend told me she had cancer. Joy because we had opened up to each other and it was a beautiful experience.

7. Caring/Helping (CH). The protagonist describes providing or receiving care, help, support, nurturance, or counseling. These accounts cannot be simply instrumental helping (e.g., a computer help desk or answering a telephone) and should contain emotional expressions of love, tenderness, warmth, or nurturance.

(*continued*)

TABLE 4.6. (*continued*)

Examples of CH

- After I was sexually assaulted, my world was torn apart. The only thing that was stable in my life was the support I received from my mother.
- I like the feeling of being a vocal advocate, and I would like to help others with similar problems.
- I held his hand to help him over the rocks safely.
- So I decided to have them settle their differences by taking them back to my room, and for the next few hours, I had them talking and explaining each other's hatred, why there were miscommunications.

8. Unity/Togetherness (UT). The protagonist experiences and expresses a sense of being part of a larger community beyond oneself. This community could range from family, a group of friends, a team or a local community to a religious order, an ethnic group, or a nation. It could also contain a sense of connection to the entire human race, the animal world, the world of nature, or a spiritual presence.

Examples of UT

- The most important part of the day was being surrounded by my peers, whom I loved. . . . I finally felt completely comfortable with my classmates. I could call them my friends.
- The bonds of sisterhood can never be broken. After a week and a half trampling around in the cold, chitchatting for sorority rush, my Rho Chi Sister Heather handed me the envelope and inside I saw it—the invitation to be a sister of Alpha Phi. . . . What this says about my personality is that I love to belong.
- This event showed me how much I cared for not only my dad but also my mother and the entire family.
- I remember when I joined the Cub Scouts. . . . The uniforms that the scouts wore were blue. I couldn't wait until I received my uniform. It made me feel important and a part of something.
- We looked up and looming next to us, literally, was the Acropolis. . . . I recall feeling both small and big in the sense of belonging to a society that was responsible for this tremendous architecture.

Note. Adapted from McAdams (2002). Copyright 2002 by Dan P. McAdams. Adapted by permission.

Dating back to Freud and Adler, researchers and clinicians have treated memories the way they treat dreams or projective tests and analyzed them for their underlying themes and motives (for reviews, see Bruhn, 1984, 1990; Singer & Salovey, 1993). More recently, researchers have proposed various systems for linking memory content to important goals, enduring concerns, and unresolved conflicts (Moffitt & Singer, 1994; Pillemer, 2001; Singer & Salovey, 1993; Tomkins, 1987; Woike, 1995; Woike et al., 1999). In an early descriptive study, Pillemer, Rhinehart, and White (1986) found that themes revolving around recreation, romance, and family life are prevalent in the autobiographical memories of students after transition to college. Core themes of interactions, motives, and wishes in autobiographical memories, scored by Luborsky's (1990) method, may predict self-esteem and its fluctuations (Thorne & Michaelieu, 1996). Scores on the agency and communion motives in the TAT narratives of participants are congruent with the thematic content of their daily memory diaries (Woike & Polo, 2001). A recent method of scoring memories for themes of redemption and contamination yielded associations with well-being and adjustment (McAdams et al., 2001).

In contrast to these thematic approaches, Thorne and McLean (2001) developed empirically a scoring system for a range of mutually exclusive types of *events* reflected in self-defining memories. Based on a series of studies, totaling nearly 1,000 memories, the *Manual for Coding Events in Self-Defining Memories* (Thorne & McLean, 2001) identifies nine major categories of memory event narratives. Narratives of *threat* are about deaths, accidents, assaults, illness, and other concerns with personal safety. (There are five subcategories: threat to someone else, accident/illness of self, physical assault to self, sexual assault to self, and not classifiable.) Narratives of *disrupted relationships* include breakup, divorce, separation, and interpersonal conflict. *Undisrupted relationships* focus on relationships without conflicts. *Achievement/mastery* narratives (e.g., winning competitions, learning skills, getting into college, becoming popular) emphasize success and end on a positive note, whereas *failure* narratives emphasize frustrated attempts at achievement and end in a negative way. Narratives of *recreation/exploration* are about play and enjoyment. *Guilt/shame* narratives revolve around the issue of doing right or wrong (e.g., remorse for stealing). *Drugs/alcohol* narratives are exclusively about substance use for recreation, thrill, or suicide. The last category is "event not classifiable."

Thorne et al. (2004) have found that in college student samples, relationship memories are the most prevalent, accounting for roughly 40% of the memories (they do not offer a breakdown of undisrupted vs. disrupted relationships), followed by threat (approximately 25%), leisure (approximately 15%), and achievement memories (approximately 10–15%). Jennifer's case reveals that she has three undisrupted relationship memories (the Florida trip with mother, the family cruise, and climbing in the crib with brother), two disrupted relationship memories (high school graduation and being dropped off at college), one threat memory (death of her grandfather), and two achievement-oriented memories (deciding to join a figure-skating club; deciding to join the soccer team). She also has two memories that are not easily classifiable (beginning to feel negatively about herself; transferring to new college). Of the eight classifiable memories, we can note that six memories make reference to relationships with family members, while the other two convey ambivalence about achievement/mastery situations. Confirming an earlier finding from our analysis of Jennifer's personal strivings, it is particularly remarkable that none of her memories mention a specific friend or romantic relationship. Though she mentions leaving friends from high school behind when she graduated and adjusting socially after her transfer to a new college, she has nothing more particular to say about any relationship outside her family. Having scored several hundred 10-memory protocols over the years, I can attest to the extreme poverty of peer intimacy expressed in Jennifer's set of 10 memories. The usual protocol of memories is filled with reference to other peers (friends and rivals), as well as a strong presence of romantic partners.

MEMORY THEMES

Turning from the memories' literal content to their thematic coding, we can rely on Dan McAdams's (2002) *Coding Autobiographical Episodes for Themes of Agency and Communion* (most recently revised on October 17, 2002; see Appendix A and Table 4.6). This system allows one to code any autobiographical episode (e.g., self-defining memory, turning point memory, earliest memory, most significant memory, etc.) for themes of Agency and Communion. Agency themes, as discussed earlier in this chapter, capture a concern with independence, achievement, power, control, and separation. As McAdams notes in his coding system, these themes are relatively normative for most Western-reared individuals, and it is highly likely that memories about self-definition or turning points will make reference to instances of achievement triumph or increasing autonomy and self-mastery. However, he has designed his scoring for agency to target statements that are more extreme in their expression of unusual accomplishments or autonomy. In contrast, Communion themes fundamentally express connection among individuals and their coming together in intimate, affectionate, and nurturing ways. Themes of love, friendship, helping, and sharing, and the positive emotions associated with these themes, are all critical to the communal coding category.

As Table 4.6 displays, there are eight different themes: four agentic and four communal in the scoring system. The four agency themes consist of (1) Achievement/Responsibility (AR), (2) Power/Impact (PI), (3) Self-Insight (SI), and (4) Status/Victory (SV). The four communion themes consist of (5) Love/Friendship, (6) Dialogue (DG), (7) Caring/Help (CH), and (8) Unity/Togetherness (UT). Each theme is only scored once per memory and allocated a simple 0 or 1, so the maximum total score for either agency or communion would be 4 for a given memory.

In comparison to the more broad content scoring system employed by Thorne and McLean (2001), the thematic coding system is more strictly focused and requires explicit language that corresponds to the exact thematic emphasis defined by each of the eight subcategories. Whenever possible, it is best to have two independent raters score the memories and to ensure that they are well trained before their scoring is compared for interrater reliability.

Using the McAdams coding system (2002) for scoring Agency and Communion in Jennifer's memories, we obtained a 0 score for Agency and a score of 3 for Communion. The Florida trip with her mother, the family cruise, and climbing into her brother's crib all convey Jennifer's commitment to coming together with her family (in fact, all three memories have the word *together* in them). Interestingly, in comparing the stricter thematic criteria of McAdams's system versus the literal content system of Thorne and McLean (2001), the two achievement memories (deciding to join the figure-skating club, and deciding to play soccer at her new college) no longer receive a positive score for agentic achievement. McAdams's thematic system allows us to measure the intensity of the agentic motive, not simply the mere mention of an achievement ex perience. In Jennifer's case, although she mentions two competitive areas, skating and soccer, she does not express any sense of accomplishment/ mastery or status/victory regarding these endeavors. In fact, her lack of commentary on the outcome of these challenges is perhaps the most striking aspect of these memories. The figure-skating memory ends with "It was a huge commitment and one that changed my adolescent years," while her soccer memory concludes, "I decided to challenge myself and play." Both memories make no further statement about the success or failure of her efforts in these sports.

MEMORY SCRIPT

A thematic analysis, then, points us in the same direction as earlier motive-relevant scoring, whether toward Jennifer's high Agreeableness and low Conscientiousness on the NEO PI-R or her high Affiliation and low Achievement and Power scores on her Personal Strivings. However, this Domain 3 analysis offers an additional narrative element to ponder. By looking at how Jennifer structures the stories of her remembered experiences, we begin to gain additional insight into how she is currently constructing and organizing her sense of identity.

Our analysis of narrative structure and integrative meaning illustrates how Jennifer seems to stop short of looking more deeply at and resolving the ambivalences in her life. She keeps her memories at a level of generality that protects her from specific imagery that might cause her to relive and feel more deeply these important moments from her past. Simultaneously, she is either incapable or unwilling to extract meaning from these past experiences—to draw insights or lessons that might guide her into more adaptive or effective courses of action. Accessing neither the emotional nor the cognitive information offered from memory, she is likely to face substantial difficulty in making decisions about how to act in current and future situations. This dilemma is expressed most powerfully in the content and themes of Jennifer's narrative memories. Looking at her memories again in Table 4.4, we can see how even her most important memory—the death of her grandfather—has no statements of emotion or meaning in its narrative. There is no resolution, simply the statement of fact that it was the first time she had lost a family member. The next memory of her transfer ends with the flat statement, ". . . it was a big adjustment." How indeed was this experience self-defining? Was it a successful adjustment? It would appear to be, given her positive rating of the memory, but Jennifer is unable to express this sentiment in her narrative. Her decision to join the figure-skating club is a "huge commitment and one that changed my adolescent years." In what way was her life changed? Here, she neglects even to circle the emotion ratings, so we can only speculate about whether she views this decision in a positive or negative fashion. Her description is vacant of emotion and interpretation.

The next memory, the family cruise, takes a more active stand: "It brought my family closer together." But did this memory provide her some self-understanding or insight about the importance of family? Her growing insecurity (memory 5) has made life more difficult and is something that "affects me on a daily basis," but the nature of its effects is left unspecified. Presumably, it causes her pain or prevents her from taking action, or limits her plans, but she is silent on these details. Her first Florida trip with her mother, though rated very positively, evinces within the narrative no expression of emotion or conclusion about the relationship, or its subsequent deepening after the trip. Her "being dropped off at college" leaves Jennifer in a place of a new independence and not knowing anyone, but she does not conclude that she learned to overcome this dislocation, nor does she say she was overwhelmed by it. The narrative sits isolated on the page, without any context to provide its emotional and personal significance. Most mysteriously (since this was also her response to the request for her earliest memory during the Life-Story Interview), the two-sentence memory of climbing into her brother's crib follows next. Though a generic memory and not a specific moment in time, it is the most evocative and vivid of all the memories she supplied. Yet it contains no commentary on its significance in her life. Similarly, her decision to play soccer at her new college ends with "I decided to challenge myself and play," but we hear nothing of the ultimate import of this decision. And finally, her graduating high school creates the dilemma of leaving "a situation that I was comfortable in for one that was uncertain (college)." Did this transition result in a lesson learned, increased self-confidence, or a greater appreciation of what was left behind? We do not know from this narrative.

I have gone through all 10 of the memories in this fashion in order to illustrate what was identified earlier as a "script" (Demorest, 1995; Singer & Salovey, 1993; Thorne, 1995; Tomkins, 1979). As I discussed in the first part of this chapter, a script is a particular sequence of action–emotion–outcome expressed originally in a scene. Then, over time, due to repetition over multiple scenes (with minor variations), it becomes abstracted into a schematic or prototypical form. In Jennifer's case, her 10 memories demonstrate a clear coalescence around a particular sequence of *challenge–suppressed emotion–lack of resolution*. We are reminded here that her four lowest facet scores across all five dimensions of the NEO PI-R were Assertiveness, Activity, Actions, and Order. These facets all share her recognition of an inability to move herself toward resolute action and to organize her world into demarcated boundaries, limits, and endings. Only her positive family-oriented memories come to a kind of closure, but even within these memories, without exception, there is no overt statement of summary emotion or meaning making.

In the words of an old Talking Heads song, Jennifer's memories get to a certain point and then "stop making sense." With the exception of the comfort she finds burrowed into the warmth of her family, all of her other memories tend to end before they assert a feeling or deduce a meaning. Analysis at the third domain, Narrative Identity, has yielded an underlying script within Jennifer's personality that organizes and perhaps directs the experiences that define (or fail to define) her life. From our knowledge of traits and characteristic adaptations, we have learned about Jennifer's social anxiety, vulnerability to depression and stress, and dependence on her family. We have learned about her negative self-image with regard to her intelligence and appearance, which results in her eagerness to avoid criticism at all costs. We have learned about her defensive coping strategies, including an excessive agreeableness, a tendency to reaction formation that turns anger inward, and rigid commitment to familiar routines and avoidance of novelty. We have seen that these struggles with her own self-image and health have stymied Jennifer's agentic ambition on the one hand and pursuit of intimacy on the other. Yet all of this knowledge is like the background to a character, but it still leaves out the *story*—the way that Jennifer, with her unique combination of traits, strivings, and defenses, expresses these characteristics in a lived life. The script we have now identified across our memories leads us to ask: What has happened or is happening in Jennifer's life that preempts her growth or stepping forward into a more mature identity?

JENNIFER'S LIFE-STORY ANALYSIS

As the last step in efforts to find Jennifer through McAdams's three-domain framework, we employ the language of his life-story theory of identity. Based on the Life-Story Interview and Josselson's Identity Status Interview, as well as the Self-Defining Memory task, we can collect this information into a formulation that captures Jennifer's *ideological setting, thematic lines, imagoes, nuclear episodes, generativity scripts,* and *narrative complexity.*

Beginning with Jennifer's ideological setting, it is clear that she sees the world outside her family circle as threatening and uncertain. She is highly prone to expect criticism and rejection by individuals who are less tolerant and open-minded than she perceives herself to be. In contrast to her family's tolerance and acceptance, she sees her life outside the home as taking place in a hostile world.

We have spent extensive time on the thematic lines of Agency and Communion. Suffice to say that Jennifer has a strong need for connection and nurturance from family members and a small group of trusted friends. However, it would be most accurate to characterize the strength of her communal theme as being driven by affiliation rather than intimacy. She often seems more inclined to relish relationships for the comfort and support they provide rather than the pleasure and warmth they engender. Her story features highly ambivalent forays into agentic achievement, specifically in the athletic area, but offers little evidence of future-oriented agency with regard to increasing independence or vocational ambition.

Her imagoes, those prototypical characters that emerge as archetypal expressions of agentic and communal themes in the life narrative, are markedly vague and shadowy. At most, we find that her father, depicted as warm and "goofy," is the person with whom she identifies and bonds most closely. Jennifer also found security and support with her brother, first in his crib, then later at college. Together, these men in her life symbolize ports of safety in the hostile and unsettled larger world. Two other minor but intriguing symbolic characters also surface. On the one hand, there is the mentally disabled cousin, who in the innocence of her disorder, is perennially positive and upbeat about life. Despite her disability, she manages to live at home and participate in athletics and other social activities. In contrast, there is her mother's father, Jennifer's grandfather, who suffers from a severe anxiety disorder, not unlike Jennifer's ongoing concerns, and is institutionalized and severely hampered from participating in activities beyond his bedroom. These two characters play out Jennifer's tension about the role of reflection in her own life. Jennifer's cousin, due to her disability, is unable to engage in extensive introspection about her life and seems the happier for it. Her grandfather, who requires care and is institutionalized, ruminates too much about his life and suffers debilitating consequences. Finally, hovering at the periphery of her consciousness like a fuzzy and engulfing blanket, the diffuse communal imago of her relatives—uncles, aunts, cousins, grandparents—provides warmth, safety, and comfort.

We have already analyzed Jennifer's overall memories for their revelation of a nuclear script in which challenge is introduced and left unresolved, but we also have identified what may be Jennifer's key nuclear episode—her memory of her brother's crib. This memory is the most powerful candidate for a critical episode in her life, due to her choice to repeat this memory twice in her life narrative interview. She first selected it as one of her 10 self-defining memories, then recalled it again as her "earliest memory" as part of the prompts included in the Life-Story Interview. As mentioned earlier, Adler (1927, 1930; Ansbacher, 1947, 1973) argued that one's earliest memory functioned as a projective expression of one's current attitudes and most desired life goals. Jennifer's depiction of crawling into her brother's crib as her earliest memory is a statement about her current wish to find comfort with her family and escape the threatening sense of aloneness that has begun to engulf her with her imminent graduation from college.

Her transfer to a college that her brother attends and is closer to home is in some ways a concrete rendering of the desire expressed in the memory. On the other hand, as we have seen at several points across all three domains, Jennifer's choice to transfer appears to have been a positive step of assertion on her part—a statement that she will take action to improve her situation and can find greater happiness from this decision to make a decision. In other words, it is too reductionist to see Jennifer's transfer as only a retreat and a defeat of her efforts at independence. Just as her act of slipping out of her own crib and climbing up the wooden slats to plop down next to her brother is in some ways an act of defiance, it may also be that her determination to pitch her tent in the camp of her family is also a kind of declaration. She will not simply follow the normative conventions for her age group of leaving family behind to become an autonomous agent in the "production mill" of contemporary society. Only the future events of her life will shed light on the full implications, positive and negative, of her intense investment in her family life.

Such speculations about the future move us to consider how her overall story will turn out; that is, what will her generative legacy be? Is her story likely to end with a sense of contribution to others, a legacy of achievement in some area of public or community life, whether in the arts or industry, or a giving of her self in the private sphere of family, whether in child rearing, mentoring, or caretaking those younger or older than herself? As I noted, Jennifer's future is still quite clouded, but her high level of Agreeableness and her willingness to express love within her family context suggest a strong likelihood that her adult life will be characterized in one form or another by kind acts toward others and a general theme of service. The only factor that might preempt this prediction is the paralyzing effects that her tendency toward depression and anxiety have on her capacity to assert herself and take action. If she is not able to keep these "beasts" in check, she may spend her greatest energy simply battling them and lose opportunities to contribute to others' lives.

Finally, we turn to the narrative complexity of the life story and memories Jennifer has provided. In previous work (Singer & Salovey, 1993), we have linked narrative complexity to two dimensions of plot and integration. First, as McAdams (1988) has demonstrated, the number of subplots, twists and turns, and ambiguities identifiable in the narrative is correlated with individuals' stage of ego development (Loevinger, 1976). Individuals with a greater tolerance of ambivalence and an enhanced ability to step outside of themselves and evaluate experience from multiple angles are more likely to generate narratives packed with sidebars and subplots. More concrete, literal, and convention-limited individuals tend to provide narratives that stick to a central plot and line up events in a temporally consecutive fashion. As we have seen, Jennifer has chosen to record the events of her life story in a straightforward and linear manner, with little nuance or deviation from the narrative, suggesting she has not progressed to Loevinger's higher levels of ego development. Similarly, we also argued that individuals who lean toward memory narratives that are either all specific or all summary lack the important ability to integrate these two forms of memory storage into a recollection that includes both emotional experience and abstracted understanding. The blend of these two forms of knowledge captures the highest levels of ego development in which compassion and reason are interwoven. Once again, Jennifer's purely summary protocol points to this limited ego development.

INTERPRETIVE ANALYSIS
OF JENNIFER'S NARRATIVE IDENTITY

I embarked on the Domain 3 assessment of Jennifer's personality in order to place our understanding of her personality in the context of the actual events of her life and the meanings that she has applied to these events. We now have a sense of how she has constructed her life up to this point into a story—her particular narrative identity. She has given us plot points, characters, themes, and settings that distinguish her life as a unique collation of experiences shared by no one else on this planet. In what sense then, does this new knowledge take us to new ground that is different from our knowledge of her traits, strivings, and defenses?

To begin my response to this question, recognize that it is only at the third domain that we see Jennifer's life from the wider lens as a unified whole. Although I can dissect specific variables of her narrative (e.g., themes, scripts, memory structures, etc.), I am now additionally able to see Jennifer's life both as she presents it and in its entirety, with its incumbent contradictions and complexities. With the long view in place, I am also able to engage in more dynamic interpretations that would guide any further attempts I might make to understand her in even greater depth.

We may start by considering a young woman of remarkable beauty. As Jennifer's interviewer put it, "She has the kind of beauty that makes people turn their heads and stop what they are doing when she enters a room." She is also someone with athletic gifts, who was selected for special attention from an early age. For some reason, this same radiant girl grew to be an adolescent who could no longer look at herself in a mirror and fled in terror from a simple photograph. This confident, "hyperactive" child who danced, skated, leapt and tumbled for her own and others' pleasure subsequently narrowed her life to a single competitive sport by middle school and junior high. By high school, her anxiety and depression had emerged with sufficient force to require medication and counseling, as well as an accompanying diagnosis of a body dysmorphic disorder. Her subsequent transition to college continued to be rocky and unhappy but was then salvaged by a transfer to her brother's college in a smaller social environment and a location closer to her home. However, Jennifer's impending graduation from college appears to be precipitating a new wave of depression, and her future appears uncertain at the current moment.

Even more compelling than these narrative details are the few sparse but haunting images that form the fulcrum of Jennifer's narrative identity. With almost the simplicity of a fairy tale, our heroine is a beauty who will not look in the mirror—a tall and talented young woman who surrounds herself with the stuffed bears of childhood and secretly wishes that she might crawl under the downy blankets of her brother's crib. At the heart of Jennifer's story is her unwillingness to see herself as a young woman. She hates the adult body that has overtaken her; she fears the inevitable demands that romantic intimacy would ask of her. To see herself in adult terms has become merged with her greatest fear—the loss of the family intimacy that she most prizes.

Since all girls must face the metamorphosis of puberty and chuff off their childhood skins to emerge into adulthood, why has Jennifer reached an impasse in this process? What has held her back and led her to hate the very changes that signal her emergence as a unique adult? Even as we attempt to answer this question, we must recognize that our ensuing speculations take the three-domain analysis beyond simple description and into an interpretive arena. In McAdams's conception, his extensive framework is not a theory of personality. We may succeed in describing Jennifer; we may end up knowing a great deal about her, but we have not necessarily explained Jennifer and accounted for all the important conflicts and choices in her life.

Once we move to explain Jennifer, we must acknowledge our entrance into a hermeneutic circle (Dilthey, 1900/1976; Ricoeur, 1984; Schafer, 1983; Spence, 1982) in which often conflicting meaning systems battle to establish a "narrative truth" to a series of recounted events. Theories of personality reify imagined fundamental motives and then build an explanatory web of inference from this imposed foundation (Popper, 1959). Based on what we have learned about Jennifer, we could apply any number of extant personality theories to her "case material." Jungians might note the fundamental imbalance in her personality, with its overemphasis on the "persona," the face she shows to the public world, and its avoidance and neglect of her "shadow" self of desire and negative emotions. The family-oriented good girl that she strives to be will ultimately not be able to suppress the passion and anger that she holds beneath the surface. Self psychologists, working from a Kohutian framework, might key in on some form of inadequate mirroring (the irony is justified) that took place in her earliest years. Is it possible that her parents, so tightly tied to an image of the perfect family, could tolerate no acknowledgment of their own weaknesses or inadequacies? In Jennifer's words, they did everything perfectly and her depression is assuredly not their fault. Did their refusal to mirror human frailty reflect a message to Jennifer that anything less than perfection is tantamount to failure and inadequacy? Is it possible, additionally, that Jennifer's grandfather's illness may have pulled her mother's attention away from Jennifer in formative years, when she needed most the confirmation of her grandiose self from her mother? If either of these formulations has merit, then for Jennifer to look in the mirror is either to imagine the disapproving eyes of parents that accept no flaw or to feel the terror of aloneness, where one sees only one's barren form and feels no approving eyes looking back. Her parents' current overcompensating goodness and caretaking only reinforce for Jennifer her fundamental flawed nature and the neediness that she foists on all those who claim to love her.

We could go on with a variety of additional interpretations from Rogerian, Adlerian, and even Skinnerian frameworks, but perhaps this interpretive challenge is best illustrated by choosing a familiar approach that is easily accessible for most readers—a classical Freudian analysis. This approach provides us with an intrapsychic explanation that builds from the familiar motives of sex and aggression that signal subsequent anxiety and repressive defenses.

Jennifer's current "neurotic" depression and paralysis are a compromise formation born of the unconscious conflict in her psyche. In Freudian terms, Jennifer has failed to address an Electra complex and is fixated on being "Daddy's little girl." She may have generalized her erotic feelings for her father to her shared bed with her brother. These repressed sexual feelings not only compel her to stay in a little girl state (which perpetuates the gratification she can have from contact with her father) but also inhibit her from acknowledging her inevitable adult sexual features and stifled sexual desire. To be the beautiful woman that she has become would be to make possible the realization of her infantile fantasy, yet the consummation of her fantasy would clearly destroy her mother and break up her family. Her arrested maturity, her not seeing her adult self, and her wish to live again in the child's crib are all compromise solutions to the life-threatening erotic conflict that she endures. Her fixation in this Oedipal stage has inhibited the refinement of her ego defenses and blocked the emergence of a more sophisticated superego. Her low level of conscientiousness, her poor impulse control, and the disorder in her life all point to Jennifer's inability to internalize a sense of discipline and more mature purpose.

Once we start down this path, it is easy to weave even further speculation. Is it possible that her mother, despite being a "perfect mother," was pulled away from her husband due to her own father's illness, or perhaps due to her own propensity toward anxiety and depression? If so, might Jennifer's father have filled the gap in his own life by being overly attentive to his children? Might he have doted too much on Jennifer, leading her to the grandiose fantasies of union that we impute to her? If all these possibilities were to bear fruit, Jennifer's imminent return home after college would certainly signal the kind of reemergence of conflict that would throw her back into a depression. To head home, to reinhabit her own childhood bed on an indefinite basis, is to vivify her most central fantasy and fear—a situation that must release a flood of anxiety, shame, and terror.

Although this Freudian account has its own compelling logic, it is far too silent on pervasive factors in our larger culture that confront all adolescent females attempting to construct a comfortable sense of self and body as they move into adulthood. In contrast to the rather hermetically sealed intrapsychic account, a sociocultural analysis necessarily asks broader questions about the "milieu" of social pressures and media influences that shape the lives of young women like Jennifer. To explain how a condition such as "body dysmorphic disorder" develops, we need to understand the ways in which adolescent females in this society incorporate (literally) the messages of their culture. A Freudian intrapsychic approach neglects the sociocultural forces that push many girls of Jennifer's background and constitution toward idealized "little girl" bodies and ambivalence about their own sexuality. The additional pressure on gymnasts, figure-skaters, and dancers to remain small and slim increased Jennifer's vulnerability to see her height and womanly features as repugnant and worthy of self-loathing. The "normative discontent" (Rodin, Silberstein, & Striegel-Moore, 1985) fostered by the media and the heightened demands from her athletic world, along with a possible genetic vulnerability, may have been enough (without the need for inferences about Oedipal struggles) to throw Jennifer into an anxious depression. With the bombardment of destructive media images about thinness and beauty, what need do we have for elaborate speculation about a family drama hinged on taboo sexual longing and consequent self-incrimination?

In response to this cultural formulation, one might ask: How is it that Jennifer's disorder has expressed itself in the unique way that it has? Why is the fundamental theme of her narrative an effort not to look, when all others who see her feel compelled to look at her? If in truth she does not starve herself or binge (as do so many other young women with similar dynamics), how do we account for this forbearance in her? It is particularly difficult to explain this kind of individual variation when a general model of social pressure is applied. Knowing the onslaught of media images tells us nothing about the meaning of her brother's crib in Jennifer's memory or why she goes home once a week, in contrast to many of her peers, who seek to put as much distance between themselves and their parents as possible.

Ultimately, Domain 3 brings us to these interpretive challenges, but it does not resolve them. The great insight of Spence's (1982) work on "narrative truth" in relation to psychotherapy was that what ultimately matters is that patient and therapist find a coherent account of the patient's life that makes sense to both of them, or as Spence puts it, ". . . a certain experience has been captured to our satisfaction" (p. 31). When this happens in therapy, narrative truth is achieved, and it functions with a kind of reality that allows it to become the fundamental basis for an understanding of the past and subsequent future action.

Are there any criteria that we might propose to distinguish the reasonable from the poor interpretation of the single case? McAdams (2006, p. 496) has provided criteria for what constitutes a good interpretation of a single case:

1. Covers a comprehensive body of information.
2. Is simple and straightforward.
3. Is coherent and consistent.
4. Raises hypotheses that can be tested empirically.
5. Is in accord with previous empirical research.
6. Is useful.
7. Generates new ideas.

By these criteria, we might say that the proffered Freudian interpretation covers a comprehensive body of information, possesses a coherent and consistent framework, is useful in accounting for unusual aspects of Jennifer's case, and generates new ideas about the etiology of body dysmorphic disorder. Given the number of inferences required by this interpretation, it cannot in fairness be called "simple and straightforward." Additionally, its ability to raise hypotheses that can be empirically tested is problematic given its extensive supposition of unconscious processes. Similarly, although an extensive body of empirical work has supported numerous tenets of Freud's theories (Westen, 1998), no body of previous empirical research has confirmed the existence of repressed infantile erotic desires for the opposite-sex parent. In summary, there is both an interpretive attractiveness and an empirical weakness to the Freudian interpretation.

A sociocultural analysis has similar strengths and weaknesses. It covers a great deal of ground in explaining the pressures on Jennifer. Its connection to her specific difficulties is straightforward and persuasive. Its logic is consistent, but its breadth of explanation also makes it difficult to test and to apply to the particulars of Jennifer's unique life. There is a great deal of empirical support for the negative influence of media on young women's body image (Cash, 2002), which places its argument on stronger scientific ground than some of the Freudian assertions. Still, it is useful more as a cautionary tale than in its immediate implications for practical intervention for Jennifer.

In summary, both interpretations of Jennifer's story have merits and limitations. Since our knowledge of Jennifer is limited to her participation in our research project, we are forced to leave these speculative interpretations to be taken up within her own therapy, if and when she chooses to return to counseling. We can only wish her an increasing strength and confidence in herself, and ultimately an ability to recognize her own inner and outer beauty that is nurtured within, but extends beyond, the loving circle of her family. We hope that Jennifer will someday soon look at her own reflection and see an adult woman comfortably looking back.

WHAT HAVE WE LEARNED FROM THE THREE DOMAINS AND WHAT IS STILL MISSING?

Over these first three chapters, I have carried out a mission to understand Jennifer through the lens of contemporary personality research. By choice and necessity, the search for Jennifer has been highly selective, with a limited set of detecting tools and an incomplete dossier of information. What have I accomplished and what is left undone?

With regard to what has been achieved, I hope that I have provided clear demonstrations of contemporary methods of personality research that are not necessarily familiar to or part of the repertoire yet of many working therapists and students in training. I also hope I have demonstrated how these methods of research can be woven together into a unifying three-domain framework of personality. By applying this framework, I have demonstrated how one can build an increasingly comprehensive and nuanced understanding of an individual life. I started with the most fundamental building blocks of the person—descriptive traits that are likely to have their basis in the underlying temperamental disposition of the individual and in his or her most stable cognitive and socioemotional responses to the world. I moved from there to the more contextualized strivings and defenses that reflect individuals' efforts to regulate their pursuit of life goals in the context of relationships, achievement demands, developmental challenges, and particular role demands. Finally, I asked and attempted to understand how individuals make sense of their own lives through the construction of narrative identities—the stories they craft that give unity and purpose to their existence.

No matter how painstaking the efforts to find Jennifer have been through the application of the specific instruments that correspond to each of the three domains, no matter how much indeed has been learned, it is painfully obvious how much more there is still to know. In sampling from each domain, I used only a tiny portion of instruments and measures available within each of the three domains. There are numerous other personality inventories besides the NEO PI-R. There are myriad Domain 2 measures of coping, cognitive styles, defenses, self-regulation, personal concerns, and social motives that I might have used. I only scratched the surface of Jennifer's life history and narrative. At the same time, no matter how many lenses and telescopes I might have employed, each person's universe of personality carries within it a seemingly infinite set of galaxies and inscrutable black holes that threaten to defy analysis. All in all, my efforts have certainly demonstrated that even from the extremely limited contact I have had with Jennifer (less than 10 hours total and using only six different personality instruments), one can indeed learn a great deal. But what else might one want to know?

If I could meet with her more and have months or even years of contact, I certainly would want to know much more about her history with her family and friends, and her school life. I would want to know much more about her fantasy life, dreams, and more hidden desires. The nature of the research project, the fact that Jennifer was sharing information with a fellow student, and her own defenses and limited insight all combined to provide a rather limited account of her life history. The somewhat guarded nature of Jennifer's presentation of her personality only highlights the inherent flaws in personality research based on any form of self-report, whether questionnaires, interviews, or memory accounts. Understanding the whole person ultimately requires information from individuals who are not the person, as well as samples of behavior based in observation, not self-report. As I mentioned in the Introduction to this volume, contemporary personality psychology is increasingly concerned with methods of research that employ observational techniques and measurement of behavior patterns (see work by Wright & Zakriski, 2003, for excellent examples of how to measure patterns of contextualized behaviors). However, these methods are still more helpful for the understanding of research questions than for the understanding of the individual person one might encounter in psychotherapy. As a reminder once again of the limits I have set for this volume, my question pertains to the clinician more than the researcher: What else might the working therapist interested in the more or less normal range of personality seek to find out that has not been covered by the three domains?

To answer this question, I return to themes touched on lightly in the Introduction to this volume. First, as I mentioned earlier, I have left the insights and information provided by the traditional tools of personality assessment used in clinical practice (TAT, Rorschach test, intelligence testing) to the authors of other volumes (Beutler & Groth-Marnat, 2003; Butcher, 2002; Exner, 2003; Exner & Erdberg, 2002). Having assessed many individuals over the years with these tests, I once again do not mean to belittle them or slight their use. Clearly, use of these tests could provide information about cognitive–emotional style, motivation, and unconscious conflict that may not have been tapped by the personality measures I have employed. However, my goal here has been to introduce approaches that are not found in the traditional clinical assessment textbook. Similarly, in offering a person-based approach, I have distinctly left out powerful and valid assessment instruments that connect personality assessment to diagnostic categories and characterizations of psychopathology (Minnesota Multiphasic Personality Inventory [MMPI] and Millon Clinical Multiaxial Inventory). I raise the topic of these instruments here again only to remind the reader of their availability and the potential powerful contribution that they can make to clinical work.

So, given the particular constraints I have set for this volume, is there any other contribution from contemporary personality research that I might add? I believe there is, and it goes right to the heart of emerging challenges to an understanding of what constitutes a person and the narrative identity that represents that person. Contemporary personality, developmental, and clinical theorists and researchers, such as Peter Fonagy (Fonagy, Moran, Steele, Steele, & Higgitt, 1991), Kenneth Gergin (1992), Hubert Hermans (1996), Stephen Mitchell (2000), Catherine Nelson (Nelson & Fivush, 2004), Thomas Ogden (1994), Monisha Pasupathi (2001), and Avril Thorne (Thorne & Latzke, 1996), have all challenged the notion of a unitary self and have argued for the existence of the person primarily in relation to or within transaction with others. For these researchers, there is little we can say that is meaningful about the person, unless we look at that person as a self in dialogue with an other or with others. Ultimately, Jennifer's report of her self through paper-and-pencil measures or in conversation with a relatively neutral interviewer neglects the dynamic knowledge one might gain of Jennifer engaged in an active discourse with an involved other party. Through observation of Jennifer-with-other or in direct interaction with Jennifer, a critical component of Jennifer that is not available any other way will emerge. Of course, it is exactly this opportunity of transaction that is afforded by a carefully observed relational psychotherapy. What I would like to make the focus in the next chapter then is the relational personality uncovered through the dyad created in therapy. We will have to leave Jennifer behind and return to Nell in order to capture a dynamic relationship revealed through the therapeutic process.

Yet, in discussing this example from clinical practice, my goal is to demonstrate the connection back to the laboratory work of contemporary personality research and its three domains. I hope simply to stretch these boundaries to encompass the exciting advances being made in the clinical realm and relational theory. These advances help us to find the person amid the flowing stream of self and other that constitutes the most accurate rendering of what it means to live a human (and, I hope, a humane) life.

5

Relational Dynamics

In Chapter 1, I introduced the concept of a person-based psychology and argued that it blends the effort to explain personality (*erklären* science) with the effort to understand the phenomenological experience of the person (*verstehen* psychology). Thus far, our pursuit of the person has been based in the *erklären* approach that attempts to identify the various components that might accurately account for Jennifer's personality. We have quantified and coded Jennifer's responses using reliable and validated tools of personality assessment. Following the parameters adopted by the research community of academic psychology, my vantage point with regard to Jennifer has been that of the disengaged researcher, stepping back from the *subject* of my investigation with as *objective* a perspective as possible.

Yet despite my efforts at neutrality and objectivity, one could legitimately ask how successful have I been in this undertaking? Despite my efforts to describe her as a person in the most comprehensive and respectful manner possible, I think the biases that I project onto this endeavor are fairly transparent. As I systematically document Jennifer's lack of self-assertion and her anxiety over others' evaluation of her, I convey my own (and my culture's) bias for late adolescents and young adults to display increasing independence and autonomy. As I emphasize the "barrenness" of her self-description in memories characterized by limited imagery and detail, I betray my own preference for lives to be rendered in narratives rich in metaphor, pattern, and symbolism.

However, imagine that we could strip away all of my human foibles and predilections as a researcher and that the rendering of Jennifer from

our personality measurements were as mathematically precise, method-
ologically clear, and analytically objective as any scientist could hope to
achieve. Would we now have as accurate and complete a picture of
Jennifer as possible? Leaving aside the question of whether we could
ever hope to achieve a human science of such elegant detachment, my
answer is that we would be missing a crucial dimension of *understanding* Jennifer (*verstehen* psychology).

Ultimately, as thorough and as sensitive as my approach may be, it
still treats Jennifer as a "thing" to be studied rather than a volitional,
valuing person who exists in a dynamic relational and cultural context
(see Lamiell, 2003, for his discussion of William Stern's *critical per-
sonalism* approach to psychology and how Stern distinguishes the study
of the person from other "thing-like" objects of investigation). If
Jennifer is to be knowable from the disengaged stance of the personality
laboratory, we must be willing to concede that individuals can be extracted from context, placed in a kind of vacuum, and then described
comprehensively.

In the end, the Jennifer that we study in the laboratory is a partial
Jennifer, a "cultivated" Jennifer, not the Jennifer spawned and thriving
in her natural habitat. I use this metaphor of "cultivated versus natural"
in a particularly pointed way. Recently, in an effort to reduce the number
of rivers and streams that would be protected from commercial usage,
the federal government redefined the traditional method for counting the
number of salmon in our freshwater. Previously, nursery-hatched salmon,
which have different habits and survival rates than wild salmon, were
logged separately and not included in endangered species counts. Now,
in order to inflate the number of salmon present in our waters, the federal government has abolished any distinction between the two and
immediately, the problem of depleted stocks of fresh water salmon is
markedly reduced. Since the numbers look better and the regulations
that were protecting the wild salmon are now loosened, the real result is
that our true number of wild salmon will rapidly decline, masked by the
introduction of the nursery-bred salmon into our census counts. The
point of this fish tale is that there is indeed a difference between organisms in their natural embedded environments and ones that are extracted
and placed in artificial circumstances. Jennifer in her natural habitat is a
person developed and defined by her web of relationships. Accordingly,
a full understanding of the person requires methods and interpretations
that take into account the individual embedded in his or her relational
world.

My goal in this chapter is to demonstrate that just as psychotherapists can gain a more comprehensive understanding of the person by the
application of the three-domain framework I have employed to study

Jennifer, personality psychologists can benefit by incorporating models of relational dynamics into their person-based models. Since the seminal contributions of Klein (1975), Sullivan (1954), Fairbairn (1954), and Winnicott (1960/1965), there has been an emerging movement in psychology to redefine the person in terms of a relational matrix (Mitchell, 1988). "The salmon of the wild," the person that I hope to know most deeply, is an individual actively participating in a relationship with me. In the context of this ongoing relationship, I am likely to move from a "thing-like" explanation of the parts of personality to the most involved and involving understanding of the person. My stance shifts from disengaged to "engaged" and, through this engagement, new dimensions of insight and understanding are likely to emerge not only about the person with whom I engage, but inevitably also about myself.

Alas, to reach this next step in finding the person, we must bid good-bye to Jennifer, the conscientious, if somewhat reluctant, participant in our laboratory studies. We not only leave Jennifer behind, but we also step out of the personality laboratory and work our way over to the professional suite in which a therapy office might be found. There, waiting patiently all these chapters (since her introduction in Chapter 1) is Nell, the married woman in her 30s, who is battling with depressive bouts, while struggling with her ambivalence about motherhood and a career in art. Through Nell's willingness to participate in a challenging insight-oriented psychotherapy, we may indeed gain access to an additional level of understanding of the person that our three-domain individualistic framework could not provide. This understanding owes its debt to the emerging field of relational psychoanalysis, and it is to an explication of this perspective that I now turn. Based on my years of working alongside personality psychologists, I cannot assume that these researchers have extensive familiarity with the historical roots and subsequent developments in relational psychotherapy. For this reason, I begin with a historical review that helps to trace the current innovative ideas in relational psychoanalysis. I then move into an explication of these innovations, and finish with their application to my work with Nell in relational psychotherapy.

THE EMERGENCE OF
RELATIONAL PSYCHOANALYSIS

In considering the classical psychoanalytic concepts that are still taught in Introductory Psychology and Personality courses at the undergraduate level, we conjure up a picture of an intrapsychic battleground in which ongoing conflict is waged between individuals' sexual and aggressive im-

pulses, and the internalized standards of parental and societal proscrip-
tions. In the midst of this war of instinct (id) and conscience (superego),
individuals' pragmatic reality principle (ego) employs the tools of compromise and defense to restrain the expression of unacceptable desires.
No matter how many other ways Freud actually portrayed the psycho-
dynamics of personality, his theory is too often reduced to this individualistic and hydraulic model of drive reduction. Yet by the 1920s, innovative psychoanalysts who still saw themselves in a Freudian tradition
began to produce theoretical writings that proposed a markedly different
picture of psychic functioning.

Most relevant to our current concern with a relational perspective
on personality are the writings of Melanie Klein (1882–1960), a Viennese-
born psychoanalyst who spent much of her mature life in English psychoanalytic circles. As a child analyst, Klein pioneered the use of toys
and symbolic play to understand the psychological conflicts and struggles of children. As a persistent theme in their play, she detected impulses
in children to identify positive aspects of objects as "parts of themselves"
and, in contrast, to push away or define as outside of themselves negative or threatening qualities. These impulses were based in the most fundamental processes of incorporation and elimination that define the
physical world of the infant. Drawing on Freudian concepts of defense,
she highlighted the children's tendencies to "introject" and "project" in
efforts to modulate the overwhelming stimulation of internal feelings
and perceived external threats.

In particular, Klein (1975) claimed that infants experience a cavalcade
of powerful feelings with regard to the maternal caregiver—including a
desire to devour the mother as a source of all nourishment, envy of her
power, and guilt for emptying her of all of her vital energies. Such violent
emotions cause the infant to generate fantasies and images that are
threatening to more positive views of the mother. Defenses of projection
and splitting are employed to protect more positive images of the mother
from these "internalized" negative representations of the mother "object." Out of these infantile "object representations" emerge patterns of
future representations of other important, intimate figures, which in turn
influence one's actual "object relations" with these intimate others.

Leaving aside the fantastical aspects of Klein's view of the infant's
mind and her tendency to project nuanced thought processes onto the
infant's psychology, her enduring contribution was to see all of personality as grounded in relational concerns.

> The analysis of very young children has taught me that there is no in-
> stinctual urge, no anxiety situation, no mental process which does not
> involve objects, external or internal; in other words, object relations are
> at the *center* of emotional life. Furthermore, love and hatred, phantasies,

anxieties, and defences are also operative from the beginning and are *ab initio* indivisibly linked with object relations. . . . Therefore we have to go back again and again in analysis to the fluctuations between objects, loved and hated, external and internal. (Klein, 1952, cited in Chodorow, 1999, pp. 17–18; emphasis in original)

A contemporary of Klein, Donald Winnicott (1896–1971), who was both a pediatrician and a psychoanalyst, became aware of Klein's work when his analyst mentioned that he might find Klein to be of some importance to his own efforts to understand the psychological world of children (Winnicott, 1962/1965). Winnicott, who had been one of the few psychoanalysts in the British analytic world at that time actually to have firsthand experience with child patients, found Klein's ideas a revelation. As he described in his recollections of Klein (Winnicott, 1962/1965), he quickly became her student and benefited greatly from her supervision. Ultimately, Winnicott served as the analyst for one of Klein's children (Rodman, 2003), and they engaged in much dialogue and correspondence over the years.

Winnicott particularly resonated with Klein's emphasis on children's psychological difficulties that occurred earlier than the Freudian emphasis on Oedipal conflicts. However, his own theoretical and clinical work shifted from the purely intrapsychic dimension explored by Klein to the actual "environmental" conditions experienced by the infant and young child that allowed for the development of a stable ego and secure self. Winnicott (1960/1965) is responsible for highlighting the value of a safe "holding environment" created by a "good enough" mother (p. 55) who provides the necessary resources and security that foster healthy growth and gradual independence.

> The capacity to experience and hold a sense of one's own being as real depends on the mother's doing so first, mirroring back to the child who he is and what he is like. Thus, in Winnicott's system the first developmental task is the establishment of a sense of self. The caretaker must perform certain kinds of roles for this to happen, provide certain kinds of experiences. (Mitchell, 1988, p. 32)

Another British psychoanalyst, W. R. D. Fairbairn (1889–1964), took the concept of the child's need for relationship with others to the next logical step. He proposed to replace the Freudian emphasis on sex and aggression with a fundamental need for relationship that governs all human functioning.

> The basic conception . . . to which I adhere is to the effect that libido is primarily object-seeking (rather than pleasure-seeking, as in the classic theory), and that it is to disturbances in the object-relationships of the

developing ego that we must look for the ultimate origin of all psycho-
pathological conditions. (Fairbairn, 1954, p. 82)

One of Fairbairn's major contributions was to emphasize that we
are just as likely to form strong attachments to inconsistent and negative
caregivers as we are to loving and reliable ones. Since we desperately
seek connection to others, we form relationships with those people who
are available to us, even if their patterns of behavior cause us pain and
suffering. What we fear more than bad and self-defeating relationships is
the prospect of isolation in which we can find no relationship with another person. In order to preserve a sense of relationship to others, we
may engage in all kinds of defensive activities, including repression of
negative qualities of rejecting objects or the reversal of aggression toward others onto ourselves, in order to avoid actions that might destroy
or push away these critical objects.

Klein, Winnicott, and Fairbairn, along with a number of other psychoanalytic theorists and practitioners, comprised the "British School of
Object Relations," which came to have a major influence on psychoanalytic thought in the second half of the 20th century. Paralleling the shift
toward a relational emphasis in the British psychoanalysts, the American
psychiatrist, Harry Stack Sullivan (1892–1949) also argued for an approach to therapy that recognized the primacy of relationships in human
life. His "interpersonal theory of psychiatry" (Sullivan, 1953) radically
reconfigured how one might think about the infant's experience of life
and development. For Sullivan, there truly was no independent entity of
the infant, only a dyad composed of the mother and child that functioned initially as a single unit. The mother and child felt joy and anxiety
in tandem; the child's sense of comfort and safety was derived fully from
the mother's proximity and signs of her own emotional composure. The
most powerful motivating force—something to be avoided at all costs—
was to feel anxiety brought on by the mother's discomfort, frustration,
or lack of response to the child's needs. Similar to Freudian defenses, the
child learned ways of blocking and avoiding experiences of negative interaction or potential loss that might invoke strong waves of anxiety.
One of the most powerful methods of protection was "selective inatten-
tion," similar to repressive defenses that allowed the child to ignore or
fail to notice interpersonal situations that might induce anxiety.

Another strategy to reduce anxiety over abandonment or loss was
to develop certain internalized social roles or interpersonal patterns that
might keep the self connected to others. The child would strive to occupy the role of the "good me" in order to please the "good mother,"
while avoiding at all costs the "bad me" that might bring out upset or
anger in the "bad mother." These "personifications" became character-

istic ways that individuals would position them in interpersonal interactions. These protective interpersonal roles had the benefit of familiarity and predictability, even though they might not always be optimal methods of achieving effective communication or intimacy in relationships. For Sullivan, personality and, by extension, psychopathology, was simply the unique configuration of an individual's patterns of responses in various interpersonal situations. As Mitchell (1988) details, individuals might hold shifting emotions toward the roles they occupy in relationships with intimate others. At times, we might relish the efforts to be compliant and good, while at other points we might bear resentment and anger for being locked into certain circumscribed patterns required of us to please or gratify others. What is critical for this discussion is Sullivan's emphasis on the embeddedness of individuals in their relationships with significant others. Their very "self-system," to use another of Sullivan's terms, is a function of how they imagine themselves to be received and understood by others.

In therapeutic terms, the key work of the therapist and patient focused on how to uncover the imbued interpersonal patterns and distortions that individuals have built up over the years in order to ward off anxiety about abandonment and conflict in relationships. Therapy was clearly not geared toward the abreaction of sexual or aggressive drives, or the unearthing of repressed memories. Rather, it examined current interpersonal misreadings and confusions that might be directly interpreted through close analysis of the relationship between the therapist and patient. As a more contemporary practitioner working in Sullivan's tradition writes:

> Sullivan . . . thought that successful therapy did not depend on the therapist's cleverness at deciphering the secret code of the "patient," but on their shared humanness and mutual respect for the complexity and ambiguity inherent in the tangled web of human affairs. (Levenson, 1991, p. 148)

All of the interpersonally based theories developed in the mid-20th century were pointing to a similar claim—that early experiences of attachment, if not absolutely determinative of later interpersonal interaction, were at the very least highly influential in how one experienced and responded to ongoing intimate relationships. The subsequent decades have witnessed an explosion of "attachment" research that has demonstrated in both animals and humans the crucial role of social interaction for healthy development (Ainsworth, 1989; Bowlby, 1969, 1973, 1980; Harlow, 1958; Harlow & Harlow, 1962; Harlow & Zimmerman, 1959; Mahler, 1968; Main, 1983; Main, Kaplan, &

Cassidy, 1985; Stern, 1985). Harlow's groundbreaking studies showed that rhesus monkeys, when exposed to stress, would rush for comfort to cloth-covered surrogate mothers rather than seek out the wire mesh surrogates that contained their feeding bottles. These demonstrations challenged "cupboard" theories of maternal attachment, which reduced all affection to the satisfaction of even more primary "drives." Bowlby (1944, 1951), in a series of investigations across several countries, found a repeated effect: Children who had endured prolonged separations from their parents were most likely to show signs of antisocial behavior, lack of empathy and affection, and persisting hostility. These studies convinced Bowlby that maternal attachment was an evolutionarily developed fundamental need for the infant, as critical as oxygen or nourishment. Infants who engaged in behaviors that promoted strong affectional ties and attention from caregivers were likely to thrive; infants who failed to generate these bonds with caregivers were at distinct risk for continued survival.

Drawing on ethological research, Bowlby argued that children developed behavior patterns that would attempt to ensure the mother's proximity, and minimize separation and disruptions of the maternal bond. These attachment behaviors include crying, vocalizing, smiling, sucking, clinging, approaching, and following. There are also parallel fear behaviors, such as withdrawal, avoidance, and attack, that are elicited by threatened disruptions to the attachment bonds. As infants develop into young children, they increasingly identify other *attachment objects* that provide them with feelings of comfort and security. They employ the same attachment and fear behaviors in interacting with these attachment objects, in order to maximize the possibility of closeness and minimize abandonment or conflict.

Highly influenced by emerging cybernetic models applied to human functioning, Bowlby conceived of these different behaviors and their activation in response to attachment objects as operating in an overall homeostatic system; that is, individuals had various set points or ideals of attachment comfort. When discrepancies from these set points were experienced, individuals would engage their attachment or fear systems to institute behaviors that would reduce the discrepancy from the attachment set point. Borrowing from the cybernetic models, Bowlby proposed that individuals internalized abstracted patterns of these attachment dynamics; these patterns or *internal working models of attachment* were essentially mental blueprints for what individuals needed to do in order to avoid attachment threats. These working models contained assumptions, expectations, action sequences, and emotional responses that converged to express a complex, multileveled response to attachment concerns.

Subsequent research by Ainsworth (see Ainsworth et al., 1978, for a summary) on the Strange Situation clearly supported Bowlby's contention that infants would display characteristic patterns of attachment behavior, and that these responses were predictive of future relationships and overall adjustment. Main et al. (1985) employed an Adult Attachment Interview and demonstrated that early attachment models persist into adulthood and help to explain current adult behaviors in interpersonal relationships. Contemporary psychoanalysts have elaborated Bowlby's working models to argue that individuals not only possess a model of their own attachment processes but also evolve a "theory of mind" that imagines how significant others in their lives experience and understand the world (Fonagy & Target, 1996).

In their effort to understand the relational dimension of personality, Bowlby's and other attachment researchers' work took the ideas of the object relations theorists and of Sullivan one step further. As Mitchell (1988, pp. 21–28) put it, the latter theorists saw human beings as "relational by intent," and Bowlby and his compatriots advanced a view that we are "relational by design." For example, Sullivan argued that the fundamental condition of human beings is an anxious isolation that can only be managed by interaction and involvement with others. For Fairbairn, we are object *seeking*. In contrast, attachment theorists understand human nature as inherently, and not simply motivationally, social. Our natural condition is connection and not isolation. Our fundamental motivation, then, is to *preserve* relationships, not to seek out or to develop them.

This may sound like a small difference, but I think it is a crucial one for considering various models of the person and subsequent therapeutic responses. If therapists see the person in therapy as a freestanding individual who not only strives to enter relationships but also can disengage from them and return to an autonomous independence, they will respond very differently to relationship questions than therapists who see individuals as inextricably defined and expressed by the relationships in which they are immersed. I explore this precise issue in Chapter 6, this volume.

For now, we simply need to note that interpersonal and attachment models of the person had set the scene for a major conceptual shift in psychoanalytic theorizing and practice, loosely defined as *relational psychoanalysis*. A vast literature that falls under this rubric has emerged in the last 20–30 years, and I cannot possibly do justice to a comprehensive summary. Much of this literature involves arcane debates within different psychoanalytic camps that do not concern us here. Other portions are particularly focused on questions of clinical technique, including interpretation of countertransference, self-disclosure, and degrees of intimacy with patients. Pertinent to the theme of this book, which is the interface of contemporary personality psychology and a person-based psychotherapy, I now address the concepts of intersubjectivity (Stolorow & Atwood, 1992) and Ogden's "analytic third" (Ogden, 1994), clarifications of intersubjectivity offered by feminist relational psychoanalysts (Benjamin, 1990/1999; Chodorow, 1999), and Mitchell's (2000) "four modes of relationality."

STOLOROW AND ATWOOD'S INTERSUBJECTIVITY

Robert Stolorow, a psychoanalyst based in Los Angeles, and George Atwood, a Rutgers-based psychoanalyst and personality psychologist, coined the term *intersubjecivity* in a 1978 article (Stolorow, Atwood, & Ross, 1978). They characterized

> the interplay between transference and countertransference in psycho-
> analytic treatment as an *intersubjective* process of unrecognized corre-
> spondences and disparities between the patient's and analyst's respective
> worlds of experience. (Stolorow & Atwood, 1992, p. 2; emphasis
> added)

This concept of the shared and interweaving "working models" of therapist and patient seemed a natural outgrowth of the object relations, interpersonal, and attachment perspectives that had fundamentally reconfigured therapy's understanding of the person in therapy. Stolorow and Atwood were now arguing that we could no longer entertain with any credulity the notion of a neutral and disengaged therapist who offers up a blank screen for patients' projections. In contrast, they argued that there exists an "intersubjective field" with "reciprocal mutual influence" (Stolorow & Atwood, p. 3). Here in the therapeutic world was an explicit recognition of the embeddedness of individuals in what Mitchell (1988) came to call "the relational matrix."

Two critical ideas that emerge in Stolorow and Atwood's (1992) formulation of intersubjectivity are the "myth of the isolated individual mind" and the key role of emotion in relational dynamics. Stolorow and Atwood emphasized that individuals cling to a view of themselves as autonomous and isolated entities due to specific anxieties about their vulnerability to the forces of nature, social life, and the fundamental indeterminacy of human thought. First, by postulating an independent self with its own autonomous subjective world, individuals see themselves as outside the world of physical dependence and natural rhythms that include aging, decay, and death. Living within our own minds, we can imagine a disengaged consciousness and, ultimately, a spirit or soul that transcends the mortal certainties of the natural world.

Second, by clinging to a notion of our independent identity and existential "aloneness," we are able to avoid acknowledging our fundamental dependence on other human beings, and on social structures more generally, for our literal survival. To depend on others is an inherently dangerous activity, since dependence leaves open the possibility of being manipulated or exploited. By preserving the myth of separateness from both other individuals and social institutions, we retain a self-image that protects against possible domination and humiliation. We then can conceive of ourselves as entering and exiting from social relationships by our own "free will."

Third, individuals fear the disorienting nature of subjectivity itself. By endorsing the concept of an isolated mind that is able to step back and evaluate the world rationally, individuals reassure themselves that there is an "objective world" out there and that determinant principles of reality can be ascertained. This centered and objective mind can identify reassuring "truths" and can find continuity in inherited assumptions about the nature of the world. In contrast, individuals who acknowledge the pervasive subjectivity of their observations and the multiple positions from which so-called "truths" may be viewed are likely to feel the vertigo of changing postures and angles with regard to any truth.

To relinquish this commitment to the independent individual mind is also to rethink developmental models of personality that see autonomy and a high level of self-esteem as ultimate achievements of personhood (Jacobson, 1964; Kohut, 1971).

> We would replace the theory of transmuting internalization, which elevates a variant of the isolated mind to an ideal goal of development, with a conception of increasing affect integration and tolerance evolving within an ongoing intersubjective system. (Stolorow & Atwood, 1992, p. 13)

This quotation mentions affect integration, and I now turn to the concept of affect regulation in Stolorow and Atwood's framework. Drawing on the infant research of Stern (1985), the theorists claimed that a major aspect of the "child–caregiver system" is the intersubjective exchange and "attunement" of mutual emotional experiences (Stolorow & Atwood, p. 26). The caregiver both models and helps to regulate emotional experiences for the child. Borrowing from Sullivan, they see each member of the child–caregiver system absorbed in a reverberating loop of emotional shifts—a dance in which it is impossible "know the dancer from the dance."

Of great significance to their argument is how the child develops a sense of what is real versus fantasy. In traditional Freudian theory, the emergence from the symbiotic world of the parent–child dyad occurs when frustration and disappointment are experienced. Though the infant may resort to primary process fantasy to conjure up an image of the mother or the absent nipple, ultimately, the child must construct more practical solutions to loss and disappointment; hence, the evolution of the problem-solving characteristics of secondary process thought.

In contrast, Stolorow and Atwood suggest that reality is confirmed for the infant through the accurate attunement of emotional experiences with the caregiver. A shared smile, verification that a fearful response to danger was appropriate, or completion of a song with the right sound or word—each of these confirming exchanges allows the child to build a reliable and accurate view of what is stable and real in the world. Alternatively, caregivers' inconsistencies, failures to respond appropriately, or absent responses to inquiries leave children in states of confusion and anxiety about what is real or imagined, true or false, in their developing understanding of the world around them. These experiences of poor attunement, or rejected efforts at emotional attunement, may feel so threatening that they are pushed out of awareness, entering into the realms of the "dynamic" and "unvalidated" unconscious (Stolorow & Atwood, 1992, p. 33).

To bring this vision of intersubjectivity into the therapeutic arena means an acute sensitivity not only to how the patient has subjectively experienced the therapy but also to how the therapist experiences and responds to the therapeutic interactions. Levenson (1991) writes eloquently about this shared therapeutic experience:

> I do believe that Racker's (1968) warning that the "first distortion of the truth in the 'myth of the analytic situation' is that analysis is an interaction between a sick person and a healthy one" (p. 132) and Sullivan's dictum that "we are all more simply human than otherwise" (1953, p. 32) converge in a concept of psychoanalysis as a mutual respectful exploration of joint reality. (p. 172)

Building on this perspective, it is a natural progression to ask what may emerge when two subjectivities (the patient's and therapist's) are interwoven in this act of exploration. The result is indeed what Ogden has called the "analytic third." Ogden defines this emergent realm as

> the product of a unique dialectic generated by/between the separate subjectivities of analyst and analysand within the analytic setting. It is a subjectivity that seems to take on a life of its own in the interpersonal field, generated between analyst and analysand. (2004, p. 169)

In this view, both patient and therapist have independent subjective worlds that can not only exist separately but also fuse in the course of therapy in order to create a unique subjective entity—the analytic third. This third state consists of shared allusions, sensations, fantasies, and metaphors that have comingled from the unconscious worlds of each of the dyadic participants. These states of minds, feelings, images, and ideas may not be experienced by either individual as necessarily derived from his or her own current thoughts or concerns, yet these mental stimuli are indeed generated from the confluence of the two subjectivities interacting in the therapy room. Each person brings elements of past relationships, along with associated memories and fantasies, to the present relationship, but these associations are not simply imposed on the current relationship; they are mixed with each person's associations to create a unique and previously unexperienced present relationship.

> The analytic experience occurs at the cusp of the past and present, and involves a past that is being created anew (for both analyst and analysand) by means of an experience generated between analyst and analysand (i.e., within the analytic third). (Ogden, 2004, p. 178)

As a concrete example of this process, Ogden describes a therapy in which he noticed himself slipping into a kind of removed "reverie," while listening to a male patient with whom he had been working for 3 years. During this reverie, he noted associations to a letter from a colleague on his desk. The associations included the idea that the letter, which he had thought was a personal note, might in fact have been mechanically addressed and part of a bulk mailing. Simultaneous to Ogden's highly personal reflections about his own life, the patient was engaging in a rather lifeless set of free associations that seemed to be meeting the obligations of the analytic hour. Ogden continued to experience other associations emerging inside him, regarding repairing his car, the click of his answering machine, and a childhood image of reading *Charlotte's Web*. Throughout this period of reverie, he found that feelings of sadness, anxiety, anticipation (of the personal voice he would hear on the answering machine), and impatience were emerging inside him. Returning to concentrate on the content of the patient's associations, Ogden noted the patient's comments about disconnection from his wife, his brother's financial bankruptcy, and a near-miss automobile accident.

There were many other shifts in thoughts and associations that would be too lengthy to describe, but the ultimate point is that there was a shared subjective space that had been created by Ogden and his patient, and that belonged exclusively to neither person. This analytic third (as Ogden came to understand it) consisted of the emotional impasse that the therapeutic relationship had reached at that moment. This impasse consisted of a kind of "mechanical" going through the motions that yielded a mutual sense of isolation, anxiety, and sadness. There was fear that a genuine relationship had been supplanted by an "artificial" commercial exchange in which revelations and responses were simply being "mailed in" instead of truly expressed and felt. This shared space also yielded the idea that the relationship was in danger of bankruptcy with regard to its emotional yield, and that true personal contact would only come from individuals not in the room (the imagined personal phone caller). The emergent sense of loneliness was highlighted by Ogden's association to his reading of *Charlotte's Web* as a child, a book he read over and over during a period of "intense loneliness," when he had identified with Wilbur the pig as a "misfit and outcast" (2004, p. 178).

As a personality psychologist, I am proposing that therapists like Ogden are offering a remarkable insight into how we might hope to reach a full understanding of the person. Although the therapeutic relationship is a particular form of relationship—removed, asymmetrical, and defined by particular goals of insight and/or remedy, the concept of a shared intersubjective space surely extends beyond therapeutic relationships. For example, my wife may feel fear about an impending review at her work. Uncomfortable with this anxiety, she may ask me how the financing for our new house is looking, which raises in me a series of anxieties about these transactions. In response to these worries, I may have an association to a time as a child when I lost some money my parents had given to me. This sense of shame may cause me to pull back from my wife precisely at the moment that she is looking for me to reassure her that her job review will be successful. My self-preoccupation may be received as a rebuff to her, and her anxiety only increases. In such moments, we are living in an intersubjective space that belongs to both and to neither of us. Yet this intersubjective space, while in one sense unique to each and every interaction, is not without a certain predictability based on our tendency to share this space with the same intimate others over long stretches of our lives. Though this dynamic and quicksilver aspect of personality may be difficult to track, I do not see how one can map a comprehensive picture of particular individuals without capturing this component of their ongoing relational worlds.

For me, Ogden's subtle tracking of the analytic third is exactly the kind of *verstehen* psychology that brings forward the full phenomenological reality of the whole person. The challenge for a comprehensive person-based psychology is to incorporate this subtle understanding of relational dynamics into its model of the person. Thus far, relational psychoanalysis offers theoretical accounts and case study examples of this critical aspect of human beings. Ultimately, personality psychology will need to figure out methods of researching these relational dynamics that do justice to their contextual and embedded nature. Whether it is possible to bring the lens of *erklären* science on to these phenomenological dynamics is indeed both a philosophical and methodological challenge that a person-based psychology will need to face (for one effort at a partial synthesis, see Conway et al., 2004).

Having now explicated the concepts of intersubjectivity and the analytic third, I must also acknowledge the limits that relational psychoanalysts set on the intermixing of individual psyches. In different ways and with different philosophical backgrounds, two feminist psychoanalysts—Nancy Chodorow and Jessica Benjamin—have addressed the critical issue of whether individuals can still make claims for personal and private subjectivities in a world so clearly construed as relational.

Chodorow (1999), cataloguing the advances of relational psychoanalysis, as well as the significant contributions of sociology and anthropology to our understanding of the role of gender and culture in what constitutes a human life, still argues for the relevance of a psychoanalytic perspective that honors the integrity of the individual. Citing the work of the highly influential anthropologist Clifford Geertz on communities in Morocco, Bali, and Java, among many other locales, Chodorow joins with relational psychoanalysts' critique of the typical image of the isolated individual. She cautions against our tendencies to see human consciousness as

> a bounded, unique, more or less integrated motivational and cognitive universe, a dynamic center of awareness, emotion, judgment, and action organized into a distinctive whole and set contrastively against other such wholes. (1999, p. 144)

Yet at the same time that she affirms a view of humans as embedded in cultural practices and relational dynamics, Chodorow argues against either a cultural determinism or a biological determinism (the latter exemplified by a more classical psychoanalysis's emphasis on reductive motives of sex and aggression).

> Where traditional theorists of culture and personality [e.g., classical psychoanalysis] cut across cultures to retain universal assumptions about personhood, contemporary approaches do the reverse, cutting across persons to retain universal assumptions about culture. (1999, p. 188)

In Chodorow's formulation of the role of gender and culture in our lives, these factors set powerful parameters on the repertoire of choices individuals might make, but they are not fully able to explain how these choices ultimately unfold. Freud saw gender as dictating psychosexual development and leading to universalized gendered concepts such as "fear of castration" or "penis envy." Chodorow demonstrates that subsequent research and clinical observation have convincingly illustrated how such totalizing formulations of males and females fall far short of explaining the variation and complexity of any given individual. She also points out how current cultural theories end up with the same acknowledgment of the unique contribution of the individual.

> Similarly, contemporary feminism generalizes about inequality and power but points to the differences among women, as well as to the contradictory, multiple, and contextualized particularities of any one person's gendered and sexual subjectivity. . . . There is no generic femininity or masculinity derived from an unproblematic cognitive fact of gender or gender role identity, from a genitally derived concept established either in the second year or in the oedipal period, from a psychological enactment of prevailing political or cultural concepts. (1999, p. 124)

To support her position, Chodorow (1999) reviews the brilliant and prescient work of the anthropologist Jean L. Briggs, who has spent her lifetime studying the Inuit people of the Canadian Arctic (Briggs, 1970, 1998). In one extended project, Briggs (1998) made a study of the emotional development of a 3-year-old Inuit child named Chubby Maata. Closely observing the transactions of Chubby Maata with her family members and other members of her community, Briggs was able to identify a "mosaic of dilemmas" created within the socialization process of Chubby Maata that included learning language, taking on increasingly more mature responsibilities in the home, and negotiating relationships with siblings. Although each of these activities is in some sense "universal" for the human species, there were fairly specific and predictable patterns in which these developmental tasks were structured within Inuit culture. Yet, and this is the critical point for Briggs, these standard patterns were like the outlines of "dramas" that were then enacted in absolutely original and particularized ways by the specific individuals involved. There was indeterminacy or "play" built into each of these so-called "cultural" processes.

Here is one example from Briggs's work. When Chubby Maata mispronounced a word and her older sister attempted to correct her, Chubby Maata seemed to resist the correction and persisted in using the mispronounced word multiple times (whether playfully or by accident is not entirely clear). Suddenly, a standard socialization process took on a dramatic quality in which an older authority's correction was not being heeded. This brief but unsettling moment of tension was broken when

Chubby Maata's mother interrupted and told Chubby Maata to repeat some favorite baby talk words. Chubby Maata chose to comply, but then proceeded to embellish the request with even more comical baby talk. This last sound conveyed to the mother and the others that Chubby Maata could "play baby" and was therefore not simply a baby. This particular exchange ended with Chubby Maata laughingly embraced by her mother and in a sense being rewarded for her willingness to resume her appropriate cultural and familial role. Yet at the same time, her final improvisation had subtly reinforced her own free will and incipient emergence from the role of "baby" in the family, while doing so in a way that was acceptable to the group.

As Briggs performs a deep and thoughtful analysis of both the cultural and familial dynamics of this episode, her central point is that Chubby Maata's own personality and the personalities of her family members combine to make this "cultural drama" of language development a unique expression of one particular child's growth, while at the same time capturing ongoing tensions or dialectics that reflect current themes in Inuit culture. She sums up her perspective:

> The plots, the perils enter Chubby Maata's life very directly as dilemmas, problems of how to *act*. Chubby Maata wants safe and satisfying relationships and possessions, and in order to get them, she must make decisions, sometimes very difficult ones, about how to behave. In making choices, she activates the plots, imbues them with personal meaning, and thus makes them real. We may say that she *creates* personal variants of the plots that govern her parents' lives, and in so doing, she is both creating herself and being created. In her actions, culture and person actively create each other. (1998, p. 207; emphasis in original)

Thinking back to Jennifer, we can see how Jennifer's investment in a flawless appearance expresses a certain cultural drama that has infiltrated the psychology of every man and woman in American society. However, in her particular solution to this dilemma, the avoidance of mirrors and an extreme social monitoring, she has offered her unique and personally expressive variant to this plot imposed by culture.

For Chodorow (1999), then, cultural–gendered awareness and relational psychology do not abnegate a concern for the individual. Ogden (2004) ends up in the same place in discussing the projective identification processes of the analytic third. When we project our feelings or unconscious fantasies onto another person, we erase both a part of ourselves (the part that we have put in the other) and a part of the other (the part that is now inhabited by *our* thought, fear, or desire). This projective process then creates the third entity that lives in neither self nor other. Finally, the identification process allows for the return of this transformed aspect to the original person, along with a changed understanding of self and boundaries in the other person, who was the recipient of the projection. The creation of the analytic third ultimately enables the growth of each individual subjective world contained within the relational matrix. Thus, there is always the relationship, but there are also always persons who live as defined unique entities within this encompassing framework.

Jessica Benjamin (1990/1999, 1998) has elaborated on this point in helping to distinguish the difference between object relations and relational psychoanalysis. In her perspective, object relations is still an *intrapsychic* psychology (Benjamin, 1990/1999) that emphasizes the internalization and appropriation of the "other" as an "object" of the subjective self. Intersubjectivity is the complementary expression of connection to and difference from the other. In other words, we most fully become ourselves when we are most capable of accepting the subjectivity and difference of the other. Acceptance of this other person means an openness and empathy but at the same an acknowledgment that there are lacunae in understanding between two people that can never be filled. To accept the difference of the other respectfully and comprehensively is to make an equivalent request that one is ready for and deserving of a similar response. Benjamin expresses this perspective in the following passage that ends her book:

> This can only mean that the self as subject can and will allow all its voices to speak, including the voice of the other within. Owning the other within diminishes the threat of the other without so that the stranger outside is no longer identical with the strange within us—not our shadow, not a shadow over us, but a separate other whose own shadow is distinguishable in the light. (1998, p. 108)

This selective tour through the development of relational psychoanalysis has ultimately brought us back to the individual person, but with an informed difference. As Chapter 6 elaborates, I continue to assert the importance of a *person-based* psychology and psychotherapy. This person-based perspective valorizes the concept of an individual subjectivity and, in agreement with Chodorow, sees social factors, such as culture and gender, as filtered through the unique meaning-making process of the individual. On the other hand, we cannot separate individuals from the relational and social context in which they are embedded. It is impossible to understand Chubby Maata and her emotional growth from infant to girl to young woman without seeing her as part of the Inuit people and their world. It is equally impossible to see Jennifer, our

American college student, as independent of the contemporary American values and influences that form the relational context of her life.

Having sketched the basic foundations of a relational psychoanalytic perspective, I now turn to a more detailed discussion of one of the more respected applications of this approach—the late Stephen Mitchell's (1946–2000) *relationality* (Mitchell, 2000). To elaborate his theory, I first describe Mitchell's interest in the work of the earlier psychoanalytic theorist Hans Loewald, and then describe Mitchell's four modes of relationality. With this framework laid out, I finally return to Nell and demonstrate how a relational therapy would help to conceptualize her clinical case.

In acknowledging what he calls the "relational turn" (Mitchell, 2000, p. xiii), Mitchell stresses that our understanding of how two people share relational space must be at the most subtle level of experience. Drawing on Loewald's theorizing, he suggests that individuals begin life in an undifferentiated union with their mothers, their physical sensations and perceptual worlds merged with the sensory processing of their caregiver. Rather than see this primary process world as a Jamesian "buzzing blooming confusion," Loewald depicts it as a rich nexus of communication between child and parent of emotion, sensation, movement, and thought in a language not dependent on words or logical structure. Furthermore, as the needs of the child become more complex and secondary process or more abstract communication develops, this first co-created and coexperienced language does not vanish, but lingers in the interstices of the secondary verbal language, shading all subsequent forms of interaction.

As the recent work of Nelson and Fivush (2004) on the development of autobiographical memory has illustrated, our emerging memories through childhood increasingly rely on narrative construction, assisted by the linguistic structures provided by our caregivers. We learn to organize events in temporal and causal sequences; we begin to attribute motivations and rely on memories to explain the outcome of events. These narrative memories are vehicles of socialization that help us to pursue functional goals and solve the various problems that daily living presents to us. Yet at the same time, the imagery of memory—its perceptual quality—returns us briefly, evanescently, from the present to the "present of the past." The very act of remembering both announces our separation from the merged primary process now lost and returns us, with its subtle invocation of image and emotion, to those displaced moments. As I suggested in the discussion of self-defining memories in Chapter 4, as well as in other writings (e.g., Conway et al., 2004), such personally significant and thematic memories are examples of remembered experiences in which semantic knowledge and emotional imagery are combined to yield the most comprehensive form of communication for the self and others. For this reason, these memories provide critical information not only for understanding the person but also for making sense of self–other interactions within the therapeutic relationship. Loewald referred to this type of memory as "poignant remembering" (Loewald, 1978, cited in Mitchell, 2000, p. 45) in which memories yield perceptions that reverberate like echoes.

> As we become absorbed in such memories not only do we lose, as we say, the sense of time and space, but we tend to repeat, relive, internally, and in our imagination, what we perhaps wanted to recall as past events. . . . In all such experiences, while our rational processes may continue to operate and to articulate the material of experience, at the same time another level of mind has been touched and activated. (Loewald, 1978, pp. 66–67, cited in Mitchell, 2000, p. 46)

For Mitchell (2000), moments of relational psychoanalysis in which intersubjectivity or the analytic third occur are exactly these moments in which a co-created primary process language of relationship has been accessed and mutually experienced by patient and therapist. To attempt to make sense of these episodes, Mitchell has proposed four modes of an "interactional hierarchy" that may surface within the therapeutic relationship. In Mode 1: Nonreflective Behavior, there is a synchrony of movement, expression, and gesture. In this mode, patient and therapist repeat the mutuality of breathing, gaze, and speech rhythm that defines the co-created world of parent and child—the kind of subtle and automatic attachment behaviors highlighted by Bowlby (1969, 1973, 1980).

At the next level, Mode 2: Affect Permeability, we find the dynamic and endlessly shifting exchange of emotion between members of the dyad. Therapists need to be aware of how much the emotions that bubble up inside them may have been placed there by patients who need to release these feelings into safe containers. Once projected from patient to therapist, these emotions can be absorbed, reshaped, and identified in less threatening form by their original owners. Similarly, patients can feel the weight of their therapists' anxiety or the burden of their shame when the therapy is not going well. In the purest sense of Sullivan's term "empathic linkage" (Mitchell, 2000, p. 62), therapist and patient share the emotions that emerge in what Mitchell (p. 48) calls the "undivided room."

Mode 3: Self–Other Configurations corresponds to the kinds of scripted patterns that many theorists and researchers have highlighted as underlying not only transference in therapy but also relationships in general (Glassman & Andersen, 1999; Horowitz, 1991; Kiesler, 1996;

Luborsky & Crits-Christoph, 1998; Ogilvie & Ashmore, 1991; Singer & Singer, 1992, 1994; Tomkins, 1979). For example, Kiesler (1996), drawing on the original interpersonal circle work of Timothy Leary (1957) and later Jerry Wiggins (1982), has developed an elaborate and empirically tested system of mapping the interpersonal patterns that emerge between patient and therapist in psychotherapy. His work charts the variations of individuals' interactions according to the intersection of various levels of Dominance and Love.

As Wiggins (1982) conceptualized these dimensions, they are very much like the two fundamental motives of *agency* and *communion*, discussed at length in the Chapter 4 account of the life-story identity themes. Most relevant to Mitchell's model is Kiesler's *Impact Message Inventory* (IMI; Kiesler & Schmidt, 1993), an instrument that measures the automatic, barely conscious feelings evoked by a patient in the therapist. It measures eight dimensions of responses, organized around the interpersonal circle, ranging from pure Dominance to pure Friendliness, with variations of Hostility and Submissiveness in between. The scale uses the stem "When I am with this person, she (he) makes me feel. . . . " Kiesler sums up its purpose:

> The IMI was designed to identify and measure the distinctive and repetitive ways in which we go about negotiating our transactions with others. It was designed to measure the relatively consistent interpersonal behavior pattern of one person as experienced through the covert reactions of other persons with whom he or she interacts. (1996, p. 116)

A measure such as the IMI provides insight into the self–other patterns that characterize many patients' struggles in their intimate relationships. Drawing on a clinical example (Singer & Singer, 1992), I have described the case of Tom, a highly educated man who worked as a housecleaner. In therapy, he recalled a childhood memory from primary school in which a teacher had humiliated him in front of the class and banished him to sit in the coat closet, all for breaking a pencil she had given to him. He recalled not only the sadness of his isolation in the closet but also the comfort it gave him to be removed from the ridiculing gaze of his peers. This memory was an exemplary self-defining memory that reflected a lifelong pattern of efforts on his part to succeed in mainstream society, followed by real or perceived humiliations that then result in his withdrawal from society.

In the course of therapy, it became clear that Tom unconsciously structured situations with others that would provoke an exchange that led to an interrupted humiliation and subsequent withdrawal. He described both the shame he experienced and the pleasure he took at others' embarrassment when at a social gathering of educated professionals he would respond to a question about his occupation with a rather abrupt, "I clean houses." Similarly, in therapy, he would quickly point out that I had glanced at my watch or stifled a yawn, followed by a declaration that I must be bored with him. Early in the therapy, he kept up a pattern of late arrivals and experienced a deep sense of shame when I observed this behavior. As we grew closer in the therapy, he dismissed our deepening connection by referring to me as the "automatic hug machine."

In all of these interactions, I could feel more than a simple set of behaviors and responses carried on by two separate individuals. On the contrary, I could feel the overwhelming pull of an existing self–other scenario that we were inhabiting together, which led to repetitive interactional turns and accompanying emotions. Undoubtedly, my interactions with Tom also activated my own self–other configurations with regard to issues of shame, peer rejection, and passive–aggressive responses. With both of our self–other relational worlds converging, we were likely to perform an emergent dance of interaction that would often sweep us up and carry us forward into sequences of emotion, imagery, and thought. Only repetition and our mutual commitment to step back and process the nature of interactions that were taking place could extricate us from the particular constricting relational pattern in which we found ourselves. Mitchell (2000) notes:

> In contemporary relational technique, rigor is maintained by continual reflection upon interaction that is assumed to be inevitable and by conducting oneself in those interactions in a fashion aimed at maximizing the richness of the analytic process. . . . Analytic change is now understood as beginning in changes in the interpersonal field between patient and analyst, as new relational patterns become interactively cocreated and subsequently internalized, generating new experiences, both with others and in solitude. (p. 70)

Mode 4: Intersubjectivity brings us to the highest level of relationality in which we can experience ourselves embedded within a relational matrix yet still retaining a separate sense of subjectivity and agency. This mode of relational exchange is clearly reminiscent of Loevinger's (1976) highest stage of integrated ego development, in which both connection and individuality are cherished. In this mode of relationality, as Benjamin (1998) suggested, we have come to be most fully ourselves by accepting the fundamental otherness of those we would hope to know and allowing ourselves to be vulnerable to the mystery of their otherness. We reach the fullest measure of our potential not by achieving the greatest level of agency or autonomy, but by coming to see our parallel capacity to thrive when we are also able to surrender through relationship. When both individuals have relinquished their well-socialized defenses against this opening up to the other, intersubjective moments are likely to occur and new worlds (analytic thirds) that belong to neither person may be born. At such moments, in Mitchell's (2000, p. 66) memorable phrase, "love is in the air."

In the final section of this chapter I return to Nell, my patient, and explore how we moved at different points through Mitchell's modes of relationality. In examining these therapeutic interactions, I am arguing for both a *method* of understanding and a *content* to be understood that take us away from academic psychology's research construction of the person (as exemplified in the previous three chapters). The chapter that follows this one returns to the scientific question of how a true psychology of the person requires both these quantitative and interpretive forms of inquiry.

NELL AND THE MOUNTAIN TOP

As I discussed in Chapter 1, Nell, a young mother in her early 30s, has been prone to periodic bouts of despair while at home with her young child or late at night, when her husband and child are asleep. Our assessment of her Domain 1 traits located her as moderately high in Neuroticism (due to her depression, anxiety, and vulnerability to stress), low in Extraversion (due to her current lack of positive emotion and her low level of activity and energy), high in Openness (due to her sensitivity to feeling, her creativity, and receptiveness to new ideas and different values), very high in Agreeableness (her display of trusting, conciliatory, and altruistic behaviors), and moderate in Conscientiousness (not always following through on her intentions, not always decisive or able to plan, not overly achievement striving, but, on the other hand, highly responsible and dutiful in her obligations).

Turning to Domain 2, we know that she has strong personal strivings related to taking loving care of her daughter, being a good partner in her marriage, and living a responsible and ethical life. However, we also know that she wants to pursue her artistic interests and find a way to express her own unique voice in the world. We know too that she may use her determined efforts to be agreeable to defend against a streak of anger at authority and conventionality. Her history reflects an occasional suppressed frustration with being compliant and moments when this rebellious streak has burst forward in her choice of activities and peers.

Our knowledge of her strivings is connected to her own portrayal of her life story (Domain 3) as one in which she was raised in a rigid home with an authoritarian father. After a period of choosing a crowd that was the antithesis of her father's preferences, she went through the trauma of narrowly escaping a sexual assault during a high school party. This incident precipitated a period of heavy pot and alcohol use, and a virtual exclusion of any men from her life. Only after leaving her home, during her college years, did Nell begin to go out with men again, and she ultimately met her husband in her final year of school. After a number of years of living together, while he attended law school and she worked in various jobs, including managing a frame shop, their daughter was born. She took on her role as mother with relish and temporarily lost track of her efforts to develop her artistic work. Now, as her daughter approaches 3 years old, Nell has found herself increasingly isolated and stifled at home. With her husband immersed in his pursuit of a partnership offer and her daughter not yet ready for school, Nell feels trapped in her current position, with no real option to change it. She sees her bouts of despair as linked to this sense of inescapable responsibility.

This application of the three-domain framework presents an informative and well-developed picture of Nell. As formulated, it could certainly be the basis of a problem-solving therapy that would help Nell to find ways of asserting her needs to her husband and to relinquish some of the care for her daughter to other trusted caretakers, whether family members, neighbors, or experienced professionals (e.g., nanny or child care center). If Nell enlisted others to help with her daughter's care, the therapist would help her to explore her concerns about safety and parental responsibility, as well as her ambivalence about asserting her needs at the expense of others.

Yet a relational psychoanalytic approach would argue that these cognitive-behavioral and problem-solving constructions of Nell, while rational and highly pragmatic, miss something essential about how she moves through the world and exists in relationships. Although her outward profile fits the picture of many educated women who have had children and now desire a return to the workforce, her unique history raises obstacles to this return that other women might not experience. By applying the lens of my intersubjective experience of Nell, we gain some additional insight that might be crucial for understanding what holds her back from action and induces her sense of despair.

What is it like to be with Nell? First and foremost, to be in a room with Nell is both lovely and unnerving. She is extraordinarily attuned to me as a person, which is hardly to be expected from someone paying to have the spotlight in the room go in her direction. She notices everything about me—from the type of clothes I wear to the length of my hair, to the amount of sleep I have received the night before our meeting. If I causally mention an impending conference, she inquires about the outcome of this event the next time she sees me. Although I could simply attribute this detailed concern with me as mere transference or a temporary infatuation, there is a core of openness and generosity that strikes me as genuine and lasting. In moments when Nell reveals her continued sorrow, it is clear that she is pained not only by her own suffering but also because she fears that such statements will leave me disappointed in myself for not helping her more.

In other words, Nell has the gift of letting go of herself and filling up others with what they need. It is no wonder that her sketches reveal not only an eye that is markedly attentive to the detail and texture of surfaces but also a subtle sense of emotional coloring. Her watercolors of backyard gardens reveal intricate patterns of flowers and tufts of ornamental grasses, where tiger lily oranges and reds escape through the grasses' green–white fronds. Being with Nell is like being those flowers beneath the grass: She reminds you of your own potential for feeling even in the midst of the tangled world she shares with you.

I mentioned that it is also unnerving to be with Nell. The unnerving part is the question of where Nell goes when she opens her full heart to you. There is a way in which I cannot help but feel the imbalance of these moments of exchange—the implicit injustice in how much is given and then not taken in return. I feel sometimes that her attentiveness to others is slowly sapping her energy, making her thin frame even more willowy and frail. One day her concern for others could leave her just a wisp of self that will dissolve into the gray wave of despair that she has described to me.

Luckily, she knows this danger and is determined not to let go of herself in such a headlong way. Nell knows that for her own health, as well as for her daughter's well-being, she needs to break her pattern of self-abnegation learned long ago in deference to her commanding father. She wonders now how much she has enacted this pattern with her husband in a much more subtle way. She sees her husband as a gentle man who consistently encourages her interests and self-cultivation. However, she accepts his long hours and frequent absences without letting him know more pointedly the cost she incurs for his lack of involvement in their domestic life.

Nell and I have been discussing her continued tension over how to break free from her cycle of self-deprecation for several sessions. Though we seem to have the issue formulated effectively, little seems to be happening to move her forward, and the therapy feels a bit stymied. One morning I am stuck in traffic and misjudge the time needed to drop my child at school. By the time I arrive at my office to find Nell in my waiting room, I am 10 minutes late. She can see my harried demeanor and immediately asks if I am all right. After settling into my office, I apologize for my lateness and inform her that, if she would like, I can offer her additional time at the end of our meeting to make up for the lost minutes at the start. She assures me that this could happen to anyone and that I need not worry. She then begins to talk about her week, and I try to regroup and direct my full focus to her words.

As the session continues, I find myself still distracted by the struggle with my morning commute. I think about the fact that I will soon be adding time to my drive due to moving closer to my wife's work. I think about my daughters and their social life; I am wondering how their life will change at their new school and whether their peers will accept them. I then look down at my socks and think how Nell has commented that I only wear black socks, and I recall how self-conscious I was as a child about being teased about my clothes.

Suddenly I perk up and listen carefully to Nell as she launches into a memory from her teenage years (I sometimes wonder if Nell tells me memories because she knows that I study them in my research and wants to accommodate my interest in these self-defining moments). She is describing a weekend hike with her church youth group up a mountain in the Berkshires. The terrain was wilder than she expected, and the climb to the vista was quite arduous. When she made it to the top and looked out over the thick canopy of green hills and spotted a circling red-tailed hawk, she felt not only a surge of freedom but also a dizzying rush of thoughts, including an image of her body suspended in a free fall over the precipice. Almost faint from the mix of sensations, she started to wander back down the trail but in her addled state chose the wrong path. Within minutes, she realized that she was separated from the group, but she was not sure how to rejoin them. For the next 45 minutes, she walked deeper into the woods, unsure of the direction that she was traveling. She recalled feeling a mixture of terror and fascination at her absolute aloneness. Finally, she worked her way back into a clearing and saw a trail marker that directed her toward the base camp, where she found her group. Having spread out over the trail, no one had realized that she had been temporarily lost, and Nell decided not to mention it to anyone. The memory has remained with her as a secret all these years.

As I listen, I remember an image that I have barely ever revived in nearly three decades. I was walking to high school on a path through the woods, and suddenly a white owl burst out of a hemlock tree. In truth, I do not really know what this bird actually was—it was far too south for the snowy white owl that lives in Arctic terrain. Yet it was pure white and as perfect an owl as I had ever seen.

Despite this moment of what Ogden would call "reverie," I have been listening intently to Nell's description of her own memory. My breathing has slowed as I coordinate with the rhythm of *her* voice and breath, and then I am aware of a physical change in the room. It is a moment in my work that occurs infrequently, but it is familiar enough that I welcome it without hesitation or concern.

Nell's face and shoulders fill the room. They have expanded in the manner of a Macy's Thanksgiving Day Parade float, taking hold of every corner of the space between us, rising to and manteling the ceiling. In that instant, and just for a moment, I have vanished, and who Nell is, and most importantly, what she feels, emerges precisely through the absence of my being. Then, in a next moment, a quick exhalation occurs, and we are once again two people across a divided room—patient and therapist.

Coming back to myself, I feel the need to fill what has become an awkward silence and ask her about her memory of the mountain hike. "Do you think the memory is saying that you will be all right even when you go your own way? Maybe you can be who you want and not end up lost."

Nell replies, "Yes. I can see that [pausing and laughing], but it's still better when you are on time."

What has happened in these brief minutes of therapy, I would propose, is that we have inhabited an intersubjective space, a space in which "love is in the air," and that is filled with import for both our lives. In the synchrony of our breathing and the physical expansion of Nell's form in my perceptual field, we have entered into Mitchell's Mode 1: Nonreflective Behavior. In the reciprocity of emotion captured in the intensity of both of our vivid, self-defining memories, we have connected in Mode 2: Affective Permeability. Our interaction around my lateness, her concessions to it, and the subsequent reverberations in our exchange after her account of her memory reflect our participation in a pattern of familiar interpersonal responses (Mode 3: Self–Other Configurations). Finally, our overlapping memories and associations, and how they explicate each of our unique individual subjectivities locate us in Mode 4: Intersubjectivity.

My deep connection to Nell at this juncture in the therapy is the culmination of a shared set of thoughts, images, and fantasies that have emerged in our work. Since we have entered a relational matrix, they reveal not only Nell's particular subjectivity or mine but also how Nell and I coexist. By exploring the pregnant meanings of these intersubjective associations, I learn more about how Nell lives in her *natural* state as a person embedded in relations with others, and I learn about myself, since I am now part of this embedded network.

In the first, most literal sense, we are engaging in the standard activities of our work together: Nell is recounting a past experience and reflecting on it while I listen. Yet my "breaking of the frame" by arriving late has altered our work this day. This shift in our relationship introduces an additional layer of associations and resonant images about trust, safety, abandonment, reprisal, guilt, responsibility, and rebellion. On the surface, Nell enacts her script of attentiveness to my needs and a minimization of her own. Aware of this concession, I attempt to restore our therapeutic frame by offering additional time and expressing a concern for the imposition she has incurred. However, I then settle in and prepare to listen, colluding with her in a willingness to ignore the injury I have inflicted. Our shared space, our analytic third, is filled with the ramifications of our mutual response to my late arrival.

In Nell's memory, I find the following associations. She has been working hard in therapy, finding the ascent toward health much more arduous than she even expected. In some ways, it is a spiritual or religious pilgrimage to free herself of her despair (the climb to the top with a *church group*). At the peak, she not only experiences elation and even envisions the possibility of soaring flight but also wonders if such liberation could quickly translate into a terrifying fall, a dizzying and isolating death. These deliberations make her feel lost and at times without someone to help her find her way (*I am late to our session*). However, she learns in the memory that she can do this exploration on her own and that she can succeed. Still, to return to others and not to have them acknowledge what she has accomplished feels too private and detached (*it is better when you are on time*). She has grown tired keeping both her terror and her power a secret from others.

As Nell offers these images and associations, I have been immersed in my own reveries. I am thinking about what it means for me to change my familiar routine and comfort in order to fit some of my wife's important needs. I sense not only my resentment about this but also my pride in knowing I can give her this gift of time and convenience (*offering Nell extra time at the end of the session*). I worry about the imposition of this life change on our daughters and worry for their adjustment (*as Nell changes, will her husband and daughter accept her new patterns and routines?*). Reflecting on Nell's observation about my socks, I am suddenly back in a place of insecurity and self-doubt (*now that I have screwed up, will this attractive and sensitive woman suddenly see me as a bumbling incompetent, which was my feared self-image of childhood?*).

Nell's memory sparks my own vivid memory of the white owl in the hemlock. In locating this memory in my own life, I realize that this memory came after my first serious girlfriend had broken up with me in high school. Ironically, after some weeks of dejection, I had come into a period of great pleasure in being by myself, taking long hikes in the woods and writing with great bursts of creativity. I had associated the event of the snowy owl with these explosions of imagination and artistic excitement of that time. It was also true that I had begun walking to school only after my father had told me that he no longer wanted to drive me in the morning, because it disrupted his writing schedule during his sabbatical. He had propelled me toward a discovery of self-expression, then also placed a damper on it. As a birding enthusiast, he was the one to tell me that snowy owls do not migrate this far south. In my own life, my father has consistently played this ambivalent role of modeling creativity and imagination for me but simultaneously cautioning me about the need for practical and financially responsible activities.

By combining these various associations, Nell and I emerge with a synthetic intersubjective field that exists between us. This world contains orbiting fields of expression, inhibition, assertion and retraction, freedom, and constraint. Its textures of feelings include fear, exhilaration, joy, shame, awe, sadness, and anger. It is indeed a representative moment of the "tangled web of human affairs" that we both inhabit in our daily relationships. Most importantly, this shared world is like one of Briggs's morality plays or "dilemmas" that we have joined in as actors. Through our participation in this drama, we are learning about cultural and gendered expectations regarding power, self-assertion, and the role of art versus "responsibility" and also about each of our unique places within these larger cultural tensions. Embedded in this web of relations, we are helping each other learn how to be uniquely ourselves, both on our own and in the company of others. This lesson was beautifully expressed in Nell's remonstration to me that she can indeed find herself, but it is best when I also meet my obligations to her.

I cannot say that this particular session was a cataclysmic moment in the therapy. Nell did not go out and take a job the next week or confront her husband that day. Yet this exchange and other, similar moments did mark a gradual freeing of Nell's will in our work: She began to speak more candidly in a less conciliatory style; she expressed more of her private thoughts. Nell increasingly took up this same voice outside her work, and the waves of despair became much more infrequent. In time, she initiated serious discussions with her husband about how to structure their future to make room for her return to her art. These conversations led to changes in their routines that created more space for Nell to have time alone and to assert her own needs as well as a reexamination within her husband's life of his own balance of relationship and work.

What has this moment of intersubjective sharing taught us that

might not be learned through an application of the three-domain framework? By participating in this relational ebb and flow with Nell, I have
learned how subtly her Agreeableness can cause another person to col-
lude with her in unspoken intrusions on her autonomy. I have also seen
how she can then turn this oppression on herself (which leads to an un-
voiced despair), while simultaneously letting her frustration seep out in
passive aggression toward the person who has hurt her (her joking dig at
me). An analysis of her *in vivo* relational dynamics takes the three-
domain framework and embeds it in the crucible of actual human interaction. We see more clearly and accurately what Nell's actual experience
with other people is really like. This understanding is useful not only as
a full account of her personhood but also in the practical terms of teaching her (and me) about the maladaptive directions her patterns of interaction can take. In these two senses, the addition of a relational analysis
is instructive for both a person-based psychology and an effective psychotherapy.

I once again leave Nell as I bring this chapter to a close. In the previous three chapters, I have asked the question: What do we need know to
describe and understand the person? In this chapter, I have responded to
this question by asserting that laboratory methods that extract individuals from relational contexts cannot provide us with a full account of the
person. As a companion to the methodology of academic research, I
have offered the interpretive language of relational psychoanalysis.
Building on the theoretical premises of this approach, with its concern
for both the relational matrix and individual subjectivity within that matrix, I have presented a way of understanding Nell through an analysis
of the intersubjective field that emerged in my therapeutic relationship
with her. To make sense of this field, I temporarily laid aside my objectivity, both as researcher and a therapist, in order to extract the multi-
tude of subtle shifts in feeling and meaning that comprise our relatedness. Catching these moments is similar to the way that one sees the brief
glitter of a leaping salmon out of the corner of an eye, and then when
turning with full glance, watches only the rippling circles melt back into
the river. They are often moments out of awareness, on the periphery of
consciousness, that are traceable only by tentative and necessarily uncertain reconstruction. Yet to leave aside such insight into the person because of its evanescent and indeterminate nature would be to live only in
a divided and numbered space, where love, far from being in the air, has
vanished from our sight or, in Yeats's memorable phrase, "hid his face
amid a crowd of stars."

6

Foundations and Principles of a Person-Based Psychology and Psychotherapy

Chapters 2–5 have illustrated the fundamental content and methods of a person-based personality psychology. This content consists of an elaboration of traits, characteristic adaptations (e.g., strivings and defenses, among other potential adaptations), and narrative identity within a given person, as well as an examination of the relational context that defines that individual. With regard to method, a person-based personality psychology explicitly favors a multilevel methodology that employs self-report inventories, laboratory-based measures (such as self-defining memories), and structured life histories. In addition to these approaches, which are all amenable to quantification, Chapter 5 featured an interpretive method that draws on phenomenological analysis of symbolic and metaphorical communication among individuals.

Though I have chosen to bring together the research approach of contemporary personality psychology and the interpretive perspective of relational psychoanalysis, such a synthesis is hardly the norm in either academic or therapeutic circles. Few university-based psychology graduate programs in the United States have retained any form of psychoanalytic emphasis, and even an integrative analytic thinker like Stephen Mitchell made no reference to the personality research that formed the basis of Chapters 2–4, this volume. In contrast to this contemporary rift in approaches to the person, here I argue that a commitment to a com-

bined quantitative and interpretive methodology expresses the true spirit
and intention of Gordon Allport's (1937) original vision for a psychology of personality. Furthermore, this integrative, person-based personality psychology forms a scientific and ethical basis for the treatment of individuals in psychotherapy.

To make this argument I present a brief clinical example that demonstrates the value of treating individuals in therapy in a holistic and
person-based fashion. I then step back and trace the justification for this
approach by identifying the underlying premises that guide a person-
based understanding of the individual. In an effort to articulate these
premises, I elaborate and critique the contrasting premises of cognitive-
behavioral and biological constructions of the person. Finally, I state
more formally the principles that guide a person-based psychology and
psychotherapy. In Chapter 7, I put these principles to work through the
exposition of an actual person-based psychotherapy.

DERIVING THE NEED FOR A PERSON-BASED
PSYCHOLOGY FROM CLINICAL EXPERIENCE

Lest the historical and intellectual exposition in this chapter become too
abstract, I begin with a clinical anecdote from my practice that highlights how an interest in the full complexity of the individual is at the
heart of the way that I conduct psychotherapy. A successful businesswoman with a high public profile came to see me in therapy due to a lifelong habit of shoplifting small items from expensive stores. Her husband,
who had uncovered her caches of stolen items over the years, increasingly feared the possibility of her crimes being detected and the ensuing
scandal. She had decided to seek help but admitted that she was ambivalent about giving up these acts of theft. As we began our work, she made
it clear that a respectable doctor like myself could not possibly understand why she liked to steal or the feeling that it gave her. As I collected
her history and learned of her father's alcoholism and abusive, threatening behavior throughout her childhood, she continued to emphasize my
"squeaky clean" life and the distance between our respective worlds. She
explained how, at age 11, she stole her first lipstick off the cosmetics
counter at a department store, and a rush of power and excitement
coursed through her. Repeating these petty thefts in the subsequent
months and years, she told me, was her release and a kind of salvation
from the "insanity" of her home life. After the first couple of meetings,
she returned to the question of whether I liked her and ended a session
by joking: "Should I cancel now or wait until later in the week?"

In the next meeting (she did not cancel), she began by telling me she had contemplated switching the time due to a social engagement. She then explained that because of her rushing around, she had not given any thought to what we might discuss in our session. She then told me how angry she was with her husband for trying to be close to her when she felt withdrawn and depressed and wanted nothing to do with him. She admitted, though, that if he were to pull back from her, she would feel devastated. We sat in virtual silence for a period of time, and I prepared to take up the topic of her "resistance" again. Suddenly, she began to cry, and explained that she did not know why, but she felt overwhelmed by images of loss. She wondered why this theme had hit her; she began to speculate about what had triggered these thoughts. She mentioned an impending visit from her now elderly parents, but then brought up her own responsibility as a parent. For a moment, she contemplated what the death of a child might be like. She then returned briefly to her ambivalence about giving up her habit of shoplifting.

Following her train of thought and putting together the topics she had emphasized in previous meetings, I asked her, "Do you think you are worried that to give up taking things would be like losing that 11-year-old child who saved your life all those years ago?" Her response had much to tell me about the essence of a person-based perspective. She said simply, "What means a lot to me is that you don't see me as horrible for what I do. I could feel when you asked me your question that you are trying to understand." She went on to express her worry that I might see her as an unethical person in business and as someone who could not be trusted with financial transactions. She asked if I might be wondering how a thief could be counted on to run a company and oversee a multi-million dollar budget. I replied that her solution to one problem in her life did not mean that she solved all problems in the same way, and that what she chose to do in the past did not necessarily dictate what she might do in the future. To me, she was much more complicated than this one set of actions; in my eyes, she was not a "thief" or a "kleptomaniac," but someone who had many parts, many aspects to her story, and many possibilities.

This incident was a significant milestone in the work we did together. Building on this moment of rapport, we proceeded in the therapy, employing the tools of both insight and cognitive-behavioral techniques to help her address the change in self-understanding and behavior that she sought to achieve. However, critical to all of our work was my respect for her unique identity as a complicated individual with multiple strivings, struggling to find both connection to others and personal meaning in her life. This person-based perspective was the vital root structure for the subsequent growth that took place.

What justification in contemporary academic and clinical psychology is there for this perspective? In clinical psychology doctoral programs across the country, in psychiatric training, and in federal, state, and private guidelines for mental health services, much is said and written about symptoms, disorders, and treatment protocols. In contrast, this clinical example presents a multidomain portrayal of the person that emphasizes an integrated whole rather than a reduction to diagnoses and specific syndromes. This refusal to reduce the person to a single diagnosis or a single domain of personality is often identified with the humanistic tradition in psychology (Schneider, Bugental, & Pierson, 2001). Yet, clearly, my interest in more quantitative approaches to personality does not fit naturally with the anti-reductionism of humanistic psychology.

Ironically, Gordon Allport's effort to make the integrative synthesis that I have advocated in previous chapters was at the heart of his "invention of personality" in American psychology in the first part of the 20th century (Nicholson, 2003). This person-based personality psychology held sway over American psychology from the 1930s to the 1950s, but its "middle way" approach was eclipsed by the extreme reductionism of behaviorism and psychoanalysis on the one hand, and by the anti-experimental perspective of humanistic psychology on the other. Until recently, only a sporadic presence of a person-based psychology sought to integrate positivist and humanistic perspectives (for histories of "personological" research and assessment, see McAdams, 1997, and Wiggins, 2003). It is my hope that the preceding chapters illustrate the reemergence of an integrative, person-based personality psychology, firmly in the spirit of Allport's embrace of humanistic and experimental traditions.

What is the relevance of this integrative approach to psychotherapy? How does a commitment to a person-based psychology make a difference to the clients we treat? To make this connection between a person-based psychology and a person-based therapy, we need to see that clinical work, even when focused on techniques and outcomes, cannot avoid subscribing to a particular vision of what a *person* is. When we treat individuals, we are also teaching them how to think about and value themselves—how to set priorities in their lives, and how to conceptualize their own identities and roles in society.

This vision inevitably consists of, among other factors, one's stand toward the autonomy or freedom of individuals to make choices and take actions in their lives. It also takes a position on the "detachability" or separateness of individuals from each other and the society in which they live. For example, do we consider individuals inherently interdependent and embedded in relationship or culture (as argued in Chapter 5), or do we see individuals as self-contained agents who have the power to enter and exit from social and relational entanglements?

When Allport conceived of a person-based personality psychology nearly 70 years ago, he was also articulating his stance about what a person is and what matters most in understanding individuals. His vision, brought forward in the first standard textbook of personality (Allport, 1937), defined people as unique individuals woven into a matrix of social and relational influences. To capture their complexity, we could not reduce them to sum of scalable individual differences, in which each person took his or her position on a curve of normal variation. For Allport, what differentiated personality psychology from other disciplines in psychology was its commitment to seeing the totality of the individual within the context of a given life and culture. Given that he was writing in a time of emerging totalitarian and fascistic movements, Allport saw this stance as not only a scientific position but also an ethical one.

Though Nicholson (2003) has recently brought Allport's efforts to more general public attention, Allport's story, and more importantly, his person-based perspective, has tended to be forgotten in the rush toward cognitive and biological models of personality. In Appendix B, I offer a brief survey of Allport's personal and philosophical struggles to develop a psychology that would be true to his convictions about the way to understand and assess the individual. For my purposes in this chapter, it is enough to acknowledge again Allport's original call for a more complex science:

> The psychological study of individuality will continue in the manner of general psychology to employ experimentation. . . . It will be interested in the laws of learning and in all genetic principles, but will attempt to co-ordinate these in the nexus of individuality. It will employ critical standards of observation, avoid the impressive single instance, and profit from all other hard-earned lessons of psychological science. But the interest will be broader. It will embrace the problem of intra-individual consistency as well as inter-individual uniformities; it will not be content with the discovery of laws pertaining to the mind-in-general, but will seek also to understand the lawful tendencies of minds-in-particular. But there is no need for two disciplines. Psychology can treat both types of subjects. Its position will be stronger for having enlarged its horizons. (Allport, 1937, p. 23)

For therapists, the philosophical, ethical, and spiritual framework that we possess about the nature, potential, and meaning of a single human life subsequently colors all of our therapeutic interactions and choices. When we help clients to "self-actualize" or to get the "love you deserve," or "cease a codependent" relationship, or take medication to overcome a "biological depression," or join a 12-step group to "find a higher power," we are inevitably advancing a view about what the nature of human personality is and how it might be expected to change (and how it *should* change).

These questions about human nature are as old as the human race itself. Is the person simply one cog in a predetermined plan of nature? Is the person at the top of a hierarchy of creatures ordered and administered by a divine sovereign? Is the person a rational being with free will and "god-like" powers over the nonhuman world? Is the person at base a kind of biological machine that responds to a universal imperative to perpetuate its pool of genes? Each of these questions leads to a vision of what individuals are striving to do in life—find harmony in nature, achieve salvation, pursue personal happiness, attain self-knowledge and fulfill their potential, or underneath all these secondary motives, simply maximize the chances of genetic survival beyond their own lifetime. Depending on the framework to which one subscribes, decisions about the goals, techniques, and limits of psychotherapy will be powerfully affected. It is necessary, then, to make this framework of the person more explicit and clearly defined.

As I have stated, in Allport's genesis of personality psychology he was battling with an increasingly dominant positivist perspective on how to understand and study individuals. Facing the demands of Anglo American academic psychology to see individuals in naturalistic and atomistic units, he recruited phenomenological approaches (from German structural psychology) to argue for an integrative and holistic understanding of the individual. Similarly, he refused to see all human motivation as reducible to unconscious influences and argued for the independence of individuals' conscious will and values. His person-based psychology accordingly emerged out of a crucible of conflicting philosophical premises about where one should put one's intellectual emphasis and resources in addressing the nature of human personality.

Since the time of Allport, a rich array of social philosophers (e.g., Dreyfus, 1991; Foucault, 1977; Gadamer, 1975; Heidegger, 1962; MacIntyre, 1981; Taylor, 1989) and social scientists (e.g., Baumeister, 1986, 1987; Bruner, 1990; Cushman, 1995; Geertz, 1984; Gergen, 1991; Greenberg, 1994; Robinson, 1976; Sampson, 1988; Shweder & Bourne, 1985) have generated historical and socioculturally situated accounts of the individual that bear directly on Allport's and subsequent scholars' struggles to understand the nature of the person and to specify methods to assist that understanding. In my reading of these different thinkers, I have come to see the views of the person that are most relevant to a person-based psychology and psychotherapy as aligned along two dimensions. The first dimension is that of *free will versus determinism*.

As therapists, we are constantly making judgments about the degree to which our clients have control over the choices they make and the actions they perform. Do we see the man who goes from bad relationship to bad relationship as a "relationship addict" driven by a compulsive illness, or do we see him as someone who is capable of making better choices but fails to do so out of fear or an unacknowledged desire for rejection and self-condemnation? Do we see the withdrawn and chronically sad individual as someone with a genetically inherited biological "clinical depression" who requires lifelong medication, or as an individual who must learn certain social skills and more adaptive cognitive strategies in order to lift his or her persisting negative mood? Thinking about this same continuum in another way, do we see the person in therapy as driven by social and economic forces that reward and punish behaviors so pervasively that, unless we change these conditions, there would be little prospect of seeing any change in the unique individual? In other words, along the continuum of *free will*, individuals may be seen on one end as capable of making their own decisions and taking action in a manner that transcends either biological or environmental reductionism. On the other end, individuals only hold the illusion of acting freely, but ultimately we can reduce their actions to predictable patterns imposed by a biological and societal determinism.

The second dimension is the degree to which we perceive and treat persons as *independent versus interdependent* entities (Markus & Kitayama, 1991). By *independent*, I mean how "detachable" or "separable" from relational or societal entanglements the person is and how much he or she might be construed to have a private or "interior" personality (Geertz, 1985; Greenberg, 1994). At one extreme of this continuum, we find a notion of human nature championed by Western existential philosophy, in which individuals confront the extreme aloneness of their existence and forge a unique and highly personal "essence" in response to the alienating and isolating circumstances of human life (Yalom, 1980). At the other extreme of this continuum, we find collectivist or social-constructionist understandings of human nature that perceive individuality as a Western conceit built up out of socioeconomic pressures. We also encounter anthropological depictions of non-Western cultures in which the notion of a distinct personhood would be an utterly foreign and frankly terrifying idea (Shweder & Bourne, 1985). Let me emphasize again here that the two dimensions of free will versus determinism and independence versus interdependence function on a continuum, and not as dichotomies. Voronov and Singer (2002) were able to demonstrate that individuals from highly collectivist cultures still displayed discernible levels of individualistic orientation when closer analysis was applied to their actions. Similarly, champions of American individualism often miss seeing how historically situated and socially influenced by centuries of European thought their so-called "independence" actually is.

To simplify application of these dimensions in evaluating different perspectives on the person, I have imagined two dimensions in Figure 6.1. The vertical axis is a continuum of *free will*, in which values in the bottom quadrants move toward an extreme level of *determinism* (whether biological or environmental) at which no opportunity for free choice exists, and values in the two upper quadrants move toward an extreme level of free will, in which individuals are completely in control of and responsible for all of their decisions and actions. On the horizontal dimension, the two right quadrants move toward an extreme of *interdependence*, in which individuals are inextricable from each other and no independent entity can be detected. The two left quadrants move in the opposite direction toward *independence*, in which individuals are separable entities that can slip in and out of connections with others but are absolutely definable as unique entities. Using this graph, one can assign different locations in the two-dimensional space to differing views of the person.

With this diagram as a guide, one can compare the current dominant paradigms of psychotherapy—cognitive-behavioral and biological—with a person-based psychology in terms of how they conceive of the free will and interpersonal connectedness of the individual. My working argument is that where these perspectives locate the individual has

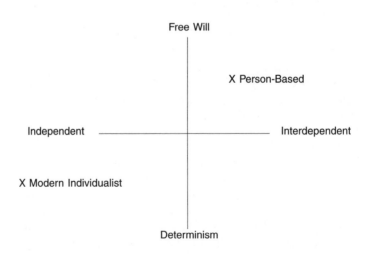

FIGURE 6.1. Locating the person on dimensions of free will and interdependence.

significant and concrete implications for the goals and methods of psychotherapy. Specifically, I see the way that cognitive-behavioral and biological treatments construct an understanding of the individual (if they are adhered to as exclusive treatment modalities) as potentially problematic for a fully humane treatment of persons in psychotherapy.

PROBLEMS IN COGNITIVE-BEHAVIORAL AND BIOLOGICAL CONCEPTIONS OF THE PERSON

When my undergraduate students begin their education in the psychology major or my graduate students embark on clinical training, they seldom ask me about the intellectual, historical, or ethical context of the fields they have chosen to enter. They are usually eager to apply the scientific knowledge base and technology of psychology to the purpose of "learning about themselves" and "helping others." In the course of taking an Introductory Psychology or a Systems of Psychotherapy seminar, they might learn in passing about the roots of psychology in philosophy and 19th-century natural sciences, as well as the emergence of psychotherapy from the medical practices of early 20th-century neurologists, psychiatrists, and child welfare clinics. They may memorize the famous 1879 date of Wundt's first psychological laboratory in Leipzig or the publication of Freud's *Interpretation of Dreams* in 1900, but these are mere facts in passing that carry little significance beyond their place in a psychology time line. For the vast majority of students (and therapists, for that matter), the immediate issues of "fixing" psychological problems and reaching insight into self-defeating patterns of behavior take precedence over the historical and social context of the discipline.

In this eagerness, we accept the dominant paradigms of medicine, neuroscience, and cognitive science as our current frameworks for thinking about persons and how to help them with psychological difficulties. In other words, when confronted with a person who expresses some form of psychological suffering, we employ terms such as *disorder, disease, illness, symptom, diagnosis, neurotransmitter deficit, chemical imbalance, dysfunction, maladaptive cognition,* and *poor self-regulation.* In turning to the empirically supported therapies, students and beginning therapists learn about treatment manuals, cognitive-behavioral guides, and mastery programs for disorders such as social phobia, anxiety, depression, bulimia, and chronic headache (Woody & Sanderson, 1998). Alternatively, individuals suffering from recurrent bouts of intense sadness or extreme volatility in emotion can be understood to require pharmacological intervention to treat diseases of the brain that result in neurotransmitter imbalances (Stahl & Munter, 1999).

In capturing this language of current psychotherapy, I do not mean to diminish the relative effectiveness of these treatment approaches, though there is some evidence that their efficacy is more limited than first heralded (see Westen & Morrison, 2001; Westen, Novotny, & Thompson-Brenner, 2004). In my mind, there is little question about the value of many of the scientific advances made by both psychiatry and psychology in the last 50 years. Any practitioner who has seen an effective course of antidepressants bring an individual back from a state of immobilizing depression, or who has employed systematic desensitization to help a client overcome a debilitating phobia, knows the power and importance of pharmacological and cognitive-behavioral techniques in psychotherapy.

I also do not intend to belittle the extraordinary broader scientific and social advances that an enlightened, liberal, individualistic perspective, based in rational inquiry and an ethos of equality and freedom, has achieved in Western civilization. From Descartes's model of scientific disengagement to Locke's pronouncement of individual rights, to the rational universe perspective of the philosophes, to the democratic principles of our nation's founding fathers, and on to the utilitarian principles of Bentham and Mill in the 19th century, one can trace a current of reason connected to a breaking down of class distinctions, persecutory superstitions, and ignorance about the natural world, combined with an increasing tolerance, social mobility, and marshaling of technology in the interest of human betterment. Taylor (1989) is devastating in his critique of the flaws of this great "Enlightenment Project," but he is also suitably respectful of the positive changes its scientific, political, and economic contributions have brought to the world stage. Ultimately, to uncouple our work as psychotherapists from a concern with science and established methods of verifying evidence would be to thrust us backward to a world of ritual and magic. At the same time, as critics of the legacy of the "rationally disengaged" individualist perspective have amply documented, the excesses of this perspective have led to the applications of technologies without sufficient moral inquiry and consequent environmental and human disasters (e.g., destruction of natural habitats, development of weapons of mass destruction, and reduction in the quality of human relationship and connection).

For our current purposes, four critical problems make the modern individualist perspective on the person problematic for psychotherapy (see its location on Figure 6.1). The first is a substitution of the part for the whole, or what I call "synecdochic" thinking. The second is a movement toward biological determinism that leads us away from an emphasis on individual meaning making and far to the bottom of the Y axis with regard to free will. The third is the reification of psychological and moral problems into "physical" problems and "genetic defects." The fourth and related problem is a refusal to see the naturalistic–mechanistic perspective itself as a moral stance, a problem linked to an excessively independent view of human beings that moves us far to the left on the X axis.

Turning to the first issue, our current emphasis on the *techniques* of therapy to treat specific problems can lead us to take parts of the person and translate them into our understanding of the whole of the person. This slippage in understanding is the scientific equivalent of the literary device of *synecdoche*. In the vocabulary of metaphorical language, a synecdoche is a form of speech that uses a part of an object or concept to represent the whole entity. For example, one might say "wheels" to talk about a car or being "chained to a desk" to refer to one's job. I am suggesting that psychology and psychotherapy run into trouble when they too sweepingly generalize this kind of synecdochic thinking. When our approach to the person becomes defined by our attention to patterns of neurotransmitters or thought–behavior sequences, a misapplication of metaphor has taken place.

At the base of this synecdochic misapplication is the extension of the biological and mechanist aspects of individuals to a comprehensive image of the person as a biological machine that functions through principles of cybernetics involving regulation, control processes, and feedback (see Chapter 3, this volume, for my own extensive use of this framework). This mechanistic view of human beings can be traced all the way back (at least in its more modern versions) to the 18th-century philosophe visions of God as a "clock maker," and the universe operating in an orderly and mechanical fashion. According to this view, psychological problems, whether emotional, cognitive, or behavioral, all involve "misalignment of the human system's regulatory components," and the therapist's responsibility is to achieve the appropriate repair of these components in order to improve the individual's "functioning" in the world. Psychological diagnosis in this framework is little different from medical or even automotive diagnosis. Therapists look for the symptoms that express an underlying disorder and once having identified the malfunctioning component engage in a series of specified (and empirically validated) treatment steps to recalibrate the individual and achieve improvement in mechanisms of cognition, affect, and behavior. What we lose in this perspective are questions about meaning. As Brian Green, the physicist and author of *The Elegant Universe*, commented in a recent radio interview with Terry Gross (Baldonado, 2004), science is excellent at "how" questions, but leaves "why" questions to other modes of human inquiry. Similarly, when we bring a car to a mechanic, we do not expect him or her to ask, "Why are you driving your car?" or "To what destinations do you intend to drive it?" Yet to divorce questions of meaning and purpose (including ethical purpose) from our work as therapists does indeed substitute the technical component for the whole.

Unfortunately, as biological models of treatment increasingly dominate psychiatry and psychology, and models of nonconscious processing flourish in cognitive science and social psychology (Banaji, 2001; Bargh, 1997), the roles of genetic determinism and automatic processing are highlighted, while an emphasis on personal agency and meaning making is diminished (Bandura, 2001). One implication of this shift is that we focus intensely on the "out of control" or "disease" aspects of behavioral problems instead of identifying and studying the aspects of individuals that express autonomy, self-control, and adaptive behavior (see Seligman, 2002, on the need for greater emphasis on positive psychology). For example, Bandura (2001) highlights 40 million smokers who have successfully quit without formal intervention. A careful study of these individuals might lead to reconsideration of how we understand the processes of addiction and substance dependence.

A second example of this mechanistic perspective with regard to the person is the increasingly actuarial approach that managed care has brought to decisions about the type, duration, and putative legitimacy of treatment practices engaged in by psychotherapists. The rationalistic and profit-maximizing–cost-reducing ethos of these health corporations makes utilitarian concerns of symptom reduction, behavioral regulation, and subjective well-being the only rubrics of treatment outcome. Outcomes that would be considered critical to a person-based psychology, such as wisdom, integration, self-understanding, purposefulness, or spiritual development, are not part of the utilitarian checklists and inquiries listed on the typical outpatient treatment report (OTR). Understandably, insurance companies are not eager to pay for "life-enhancing" or "optimizing" treatments, but if insurance companies are increasingly defining what therapy is, what happens to how we conceive of the individual who enters therapy? Does this person only become a set of symptoms or disorders?

A third difficulty associated with this naturalistic–mechanistic perspective is its translation of psychological and moral questions into a physical realm that presumes a biological determinism. For example, saying that someone has a *biological* addiction changes our understanding of substance-abusing behaviors from indicators of moral weakness or psychological conflict to evidence of physical disease (Singer, 1997). When we go on to explain the physical nature of addiction, we use analogies to a lifelong chronic physical illness, like diabetes, and talk about the body's deficits. Immediately, this language frees individuals from a sense of moral responsibility for their illness (though not from moral responsibility for pursuing and maintaining treatment for their "permanent" condition). We can now talk about a deficiency in their body that they did not create and are powerless to change, especially if the root of the deficit is a genetic inheritance. This language not only takes discussion away from personal moral concerns and free will, but it also absolves larger social structures from any moral accountability for these "biological defects." As I documented in a book about men suffering from chronic addiction (Singer, 1997), the perception of these men as simply physically afflicted absolves society from asking questions about how substance abuse also emerges from societal pressures related to poverty, war, racism, homophobia, and excessive emphasis on materialism and consumerism. Such a position is indeed biologically deterministic, while simultaneously denying the determinative role of sociopolitical factors (see Cushman, 1995, Chapter 10).

A fourth and related problem is the apparent neutrality of a naturalistic–mechanistic perspective with regard to morality. In other words, the translation of psychological issues into physical ones not only removes moral agency, but it also makes a preemptive claim to moral neutrality. When we claim that addiction is a physical illness or that depression is "organic," we not only implicate a physical basis but we also simultaneously shift our discourse from a subjective to an "objective" one that purports to bring us outside the realm of assigned moral attributes (Taylor, 1989). These "illnesses" become physical entities, part of the natural world that cannot have any normative value associated with them, in the same way that it would seem inappropriate or illogical to talk about one animal species as having less moral worth or "goodness" than another species. We can talk about preferences in the way that we think a swan is a more beautiful creature than a slug, but we would not say a swan is more virtuous than a slug. Similarly, we cannot imagine saying that depression or panic disorder are immoral conditions. In opposition to this attribution of neutrality, Taylor goes on to claim that no depiction of human characteristics can forego applying a framework of value and ethical preference to its explanations and descriptions of human interaction. To be human, he asserts, is to locate oneself within a moral space bounded by horizons of ethical preferences that impose judgments about what is good and bad in the cultural landscape we mutually inhabit. Our efforts to locate suffering or self-defeating behavior in a biological mechanistic discourse cannot purge us from the ethical valuations placed on these so-called "biological problems." Human beings can only exist within social groups, which for their functioning require standards about what leads to a valued and valid life.

Naturalistic–mechanistic approaches do in fact have built-in moral valuations about what makes for a "good life" and for a "moral" one.

These values are critically tied to certain historical and cultural trends in American society that have championed a secular affirmation of "ordinary life" (Taylor, 1989) and the pursuit of happiness in *this* world rather than a transcendent one as the expression of individual fulfillment (Bellah, Sullivan, Swidler, & Tipton, 1985). Drawing on evolutionary models, these frameworks of human functioning are infused with a value system that places rational self-interest and maximization of benefit to self and related others at a premium. We are currently in an era in which social scientists recruit neo-Darwinian evolutionary theories to explain all aspects of human behavior, from mate selection and jealousy (Buss, 1995) to language development (Pinker, 1999), to anorexia (Guisinger, 2003), and even rape (Thornhill & Palmer, 2000). The secular materialist account of human nature seems to point to no greater purpose for human beings and their social interactions than perpetuation of their particular gene pool and, by extension, the protection of others who bear some connection to the preservation of their genetic legacy. This viewpoint is without equivocation an ethical one, and it is not a coincidence that it is the current dominant ethical position in a socioeconomic era that emphasizes entrepreneurial capitalism, with the nuclear family sequestered in private homes and concerned with private interests.

In this climate, therapists are increasingly placed in the roles of "mental health managers" who apply behavioral technology to help clients maximize their self-interests and minimize self-defeating behaviors. The underlying rationale of employer-funded mental health care is the concept that therapists will enable employees to function more effectively in their workplaces (or reduce the strife and stress in their family lives, in order to free them to be better employees). The moral dictate to therapists in this case is to help individuals achieve better adjustment, regardless of the context. The therapists are then evaluated on their therapeutic efficacy in rendering these outcomes.

> The manager treats ends as given, as outside his scope; his concern is with products, unskilled labour into skilled labour, investment into profits. The therapist also treats ends as given, as outside his scope; his concern also is with technique, with effectiveness in transforming neurotic symptoms into directed energy, maladjusted individuals into well-adjusted ones. Neither manager nor therapist, in their roles as manager and therapist, do or are able to engage in moral debate. They are seen by themselves, and by those who see them with the same eyes as their own, as uncontested figures, who purport to restrict themselves to the realms in which rational agreement is possible—that is, of course from their point of view to the realm of fact, the realm of means, the realm of measurable effectiveness. (MacIntyre, 1981, p. 29)

As Cushman (1995) would say, the cultural clearing, building on this view of the person, reveals the concept of the contemporary Western person as a profit-maximizing, happiness-pursuing individual who seeks self-fulfillment in the context of love, work, leisure, and consumption. The therapist's role as behavioral manager is to increase an individual's effectiveness in meeting agentic and/or relational needs, while attempting to provide as morally neutral and nonjudgmental an environment as possible (only a minimum of moral strictures are imposed that would propel a therapist into action; e.g., danger to self or other, psychotic or extremely disorganized behavior, etc.). At its most extreme, the therapist role is to become a simple dispenser of medications or therapeutic techniques that allow individuals to pursue self-fulfillment, regardless of the moral or political implications of their actions.

Ironically, and perhaps not intuitively, psychodynamic therapies should not be excluded from this managerial perspective, though they are certainly less extreme than psychopharmacological or cognitive-behavioral approaches in stripping treatment of social or ethical context. In adopting a morally neutral stance and treating the intrapsychic conflicts of the individual as the primary medium of concern, traditional psychodynamic therapies are also prone to reinforcing the notion of the independent individual whose suffering is a personal rather than sociocultural or political struggle. The problematic nature of psychodynamic therapeutic neutrality and its efforts to create boundaries around the individual has recently received its most definitive parody to date in the depiction of Dr. Jennifer Melfi and her patient Tony Soprano on the HBO series *The Sopranos*. Dr. Melfi, an empathetic psychiatrist, worked diligently to uncover the more sensitive and humane side of Tony Soprano, the brutal mob boss. Yet during the time that he was her active patient, she adhered to the therapeutic strictures of neither challenging his line of work nor confronting him with the moral repugnancy of his criminal and violent actions. She instead worked with him to explore the childhood roots of his anxiety and relationship problems, while simultaneously providing him with antidepressant medication.

If this parody seems extreme, we must recognize that therapists in the interest of understanding and supporting the "growth" of their clients in one area will accept—sometimes on a temporary basis (see the example of the businesswoman early in this chapter) and other times more permanently—clients' behaviors that might raise in them significant moral reservations (e.g., participating in extramarital affairs, working for firms that manufacture deadly weapons or pollutants, engaging in ruthless business practices, holding prejudiced attitudes toward a race or class of people). The ultimate premise behind their neutrality is the connection of psychotherapy to science and its notion of a disengaged objectivity that does not impose moral meaning or teleological purposes on the workings of natural processes (we can trace this concept of science all the way back to Francis Bacon's 16th-century rejection of Aristotelian notions of "final causes" or underlying meaning or purpose behind natural phenomena). Scientists and scientist-practitioners of therapy seek objective truths and underlying laws of the natural world, and it is for other entities of the society (e.g., religious bodies, community groups, and governmental agencies) to assign normative and moral values to the information they discover.

As therapists, if we treat our patients as autonomous entities in pursuit of self-fulfillment, without placing these treatment activities in a larger moral–political context, we may indeed be behaving like managers who fulfill an implicit moral end of cultivating compliance to the existing social order (Greenberg, 1995). "Healthier" individuals are likely to resume their cycle of productivity within the workforce or the domestic arena without questioning the ends of these activities. Additionally, more self-fulfilled or "actualized" autonomous individuals have learned in our society to express their individuality through a variety of lifestyle and commodity preferences that, while putatively defining their sense of uniqueness, contribute to the consumption-driven economy (Cushman, 1995). Alternatively, individuals who learn to "focus more on relationships," "manage their stress," or "cultivate their spiritual side" may mistakenly see only their individualized and personal shortcomings when they should be detecting larger political and economic problems endemic to our particular culture.

In summary, this modern individualist conception of the person in therapy is an oddly deterministic and singularly detached image of human nature. Human nature is increasingly portrayed as determined by evolutionary, genetic, and mechanistic factors over which we have little control. Simultaneously, human action is shaped in a world of emotive personal preferences, decontextualized from larger social and political membership. Individuals who display difficulties in adjusting to this world are treated by behavioral managers, who work in a similarly decontextualized, quasi-scientific neutrality that buffers them from interdependent responsibilities to a larger moral or spiritual order. In the two-dimensional matrix of free will/determinism and independence/interdependence, this modern individualistic picture of the person in therapy locates the individual in the far left of the lower quadrant—paradoxically, a biologically determined and socially isolated version of the person. Is it any wonder that alienation is a daily experience for so many contemporary individuals and therapists?

A PERSON-BASED PSYCHOTHERAPY

What then does a person-based personality psychology have to offer in these disputes about the nature of the individual? From the very phrase that describes it, *person-based*, we can see that this perspective aligns itself with a liberal individualist tradition of Western society that recognizes the integrity and inherent dignity of each individual person. However, as we have seen in the preceding chapters on life stories and relational psychotherapy, a person-based perspective is unable to endorse a view of individuals as fully self-contained or detachable from the sociopolitical or relational contexts in which they live. Similarly, we cannot ignore or escape certain biological parameters of temperament, vulnerability, and strength. As demonstrated through our discussion of traits in Chapter 2, the course of individuals' progress through life is in part determined by the trait structure that begins early and remains stable over the life course. However, these characteristics display great latitude in how they are expressed and are not impervious to alteration.

I propose that a person-based approach is the "middle way" or compromise position within these two dimensions of free will/determinism and independence/interdependence (see Figure 6.1). Person-based psychology offers a vision of the person in psychotherapy that encompasses cultural and biological influences, as well as the capacity for free choice and autonomy. It also recognizes simultaneously the uniqueness of the individual and the unavoidable fact of interdependent webs of relation. Immediately, one can accuse this position in the middle of being nothing more than a muddle—an ecumenical mishmash or an eclectic grab bag. Whatever term we might want to use, the point would be the same—that by attempting to reconcile contradictory perspectives into an integrative perspective, we end up with a logically contradictory and substantively meaningless view of the person.

My answer to this legitimate concern is that the complex position that person-based psychologists advocate is the one that comes closer to the most realistic depiction of what our clients in psychotherapy are actually like. I would rather make the error of describing too much about the people with whom I work, of granting them too much of the benefit of the doubt with regard to their capacity for free will, than of reducing them to self-interest maximizers fueled by shifting levels of neurochemicals in their brains.

In taking this stand, I realize that I am pitching my tent with a tradition of non-reductionism that goes all the way back to Socrates's arguments in the dialogues of Plato. For example, in *Phaedo*, Socrates, during his imprisonment for challenging the orthodox strictures of society, confronts the premises of the "physicalists," who attempt to explain all human activity as purely the function of natural and physical processes. In their view, Socrates sits in his cell "because my body is made of bones and muscles," and this combination of living material has contorted in the proper way to allow him to take respite from standing (Plato, in *Phaedo*, 97D–99D, 1953, pp. 455–456). In this same view, this combination of bone and muscle should have conveyed his body to safety at the first warning that he might be jailed. However, he has been imprisoned and has chosen to accept his imprisonment on the basis of the state's and his own conflicting ideas about what is right. The fact that his body conveyed him to the cell and allows him to sit there is an accurate but unimportant digression from the realm of meaning in which the critical ideas that define human life are expressed and debated.

We return here to the central themes of person-based psychology that I touched on in Chapter 1. The kind of personality psychology that guides this book is one that places an emphasis on more than mechanistic–causal or *erklären* accounts of human beings (to use Dilthey's [1976] language). Without abandoning an interest in these causal dynamics, its ultimate commitment is to a concern with meaning and intention, or a *verstehen* knowledge that seeks *understanding* of the person (see also Churchill & Wertz, 2001; Wertz, 2001). In a tradition dating from Renaissance humanism (Robinson, 1976), through Rousseau's anti-Lockean view of the individual to the Romantic conception of the person, carried forward by the German phenomenologists and structuralists, and then conceptualized by Allport and Murray in the United States, a person-based psychology ultimately embraces what Taylor (1989) has called romantic expressivism:

> Romantic expressivism arises in protest against the Enlightenment ideal of disengaged instrumental reason and the forms of moral and social life that flow from this: a one dimensional hedonism and atomism. The protest continues throughout the nineteenth century in different forms, and it becomes ever more relevant as society is transformed by capitalist industrialism in a more and more atomist and instrumental direction. The charge against this way of being is that it fragments human life: dividing it into disconnected departments, like reason and feeling; dividing us from nature; dividing us from each other. . . . It is also accused of reducing or occluding meaning: life is seen as one-dimensionally as the pursuit of homogenous pleasure; no goal stands out as being of higher significance. (p. 413)

Yet, as Chapters 2 through 5 have demonstrated, the approach of a person-based personality psychology is not an antiempirical or antiexperimental perspective. Although valuing an integrative, holistic, and socioculturally situated understanding of the person, a person-based perspective clearly argues for an inclusion of the methods and precision of science.

What then might be some foundational principles for a person-based psychology and psychotherapy? Allport's original personality psychology was an early 20th-century response that argued for the retention of a romantic–humanistic position in the face of the overwhelming momentum of the naturalistic–mechanistic movement in psychology, typified most powerfully by physiological psychology and behaviorism. A 21st-century person-based psychology expresses the continuing struggle of humanistic, social-constructionist, and narrative-oriented personality psychologists to maintain a niche in psychology between the twin pillars of neuroscience and cognitive psychology (which replaced the mechanical metaphors of behaviorism with models drawn from computers).

In endorsing this person-based approach, I present the following assertions that articulate the research and clinical perspective I have attempted to exemplify in the preceding chapters:

1. The person, as opposed to a construct, mechanism, or disorder, should be the focus of understanding. Persons are best understood when their sociocultural and relational contexts are taken into account.
2. Personality may be understood as a set of interrelated systems that form an integrated and distinctive whole.
3. The person seeks a life of meaning and purpose, and recruits the systems of personality toward this end.
4. A defining aspect of what makes up a person is the capacity to make free choices and to accept responsibility for these choices.
5. The study of narrative is central to an understanding of the person and that person's sociocultural context.
6. An understanding of the person is best achieved through a combination of quantitative, qualitative, and interpretive methods.

These assertions, which lie behind the framework of personality that I have employed in Chapters 2–5, contain a series of assumptions about the nature of the person with whom I engage in psychotherapy.

I assume that every individual, to paraphrase Henry Murray (1938), is in certain respects like all other persons, like some other persons, and like no other person. There exists a unique core to each person, which I do my best to honor in my work.

I assume that individuals possess a "personality," which means, in addition to displaying patterns of behaviors, they possess patterns of thoughts, emotions, memories, dreams, goals, and so forth, that are relatively stable and can be associated with the "interior" of the individual. This assumption accepts the idea of what J. L. Singer (1984) has called the "private personality," an interior world accessible to each person's own consciousness and to no one else's.

I assume that these various patterns of behavior and internal states constitute an integrated whole that is part of a bounded and distinct organism that is separable from other similar organisms. This assumption further holds that the various systems within this organism are organized hierarchically and rely on communication and feedback among subsystems (Carver & Scheier, 1998; Singer, 1995).

I assume that the person seeks to employ this integrated system of personality toward life goals that give meaning and purpose to existence. Without a sense of meaning or purpose, individuals drift into destructive courses of action that ultimately hurt both themselves and others (Frankl, 1963; Singer, 1997; Yalom, 1980).

I assume that the main cultural mechanism in Western culture for organizing and infusing life with meaning and purpose is narrative and story making. I further assume that these stories emerge from a cultural and interpersonal matrix that serves to develop and guide our sense of identity (Bruner, 1990; McAdams, 2001; Singer, 2004b; Singer & Blagov, 2004b; Singer & Salovey, 1993).

The combination of these assertions and assumptions leads to the premise, increasingly supported by empirical evidence, that in order to achieve a full depiction of the individual, we must study how modern Western individuals seek to create lives that provide a sense of unity and purpose—in other words, a sense of identity (Baumeister, 1986; Erikson, 1959, 1963; McAdams, 1987). This identity is organized around a goal hierarchy that results in a sequence of goal-directed actions (Singer, 1995). These goals and actions are subsumed by two overarching concerns of establishing continuity with others who share one's social world (communion), while at the same time differentiating oneself from others in order to define one's sense of uniqueness and distinctness within this same social context (agency) (Baumeister, 1986; Kiesler, 1996; McAdams, 1987).

These twin concerns for finding meaning may be the specific preoccupations of contemporary Western individuals, but the effort to construct a sense of meaning and purpose out of one's life is proposed to be a universal and definitional feature of human nature. As far as the social sciences have been able to ascertain, all human societies contain symbol systems, rituals, and some form of transcendent entity that provide explanatory and teleological frameworks for the participants' daily lives and social interactions. It does not seem possible to describe human personality without reference to the symbol-making aspects of human thought (e.g., metaphors, dreams, memories, daydreams, and fantasies). Yet, since all of these aspects of the private personality (Singer & Kolligian, 1987) cannot be removed from the inherently interpersonal world of human life, they must also be studied with reference to relational contexts and interpersonal implications. The combination of concern for both private and interpersonal aspects of the self has yielded a burgeoning interest in the study of narratives as the nexus of these two domains of personality.

Sarbin (1986) has called narrative the "root metaphor" of psychology. Individuals' stories and narrative memories reflect their unique efforts to make meaning from experience, while simultaneously drawing on the extant cultural structures of myth, media, ideology, and literature that provide templates for the crafting of these personal narratives. The systematic study of narrative identity (Singer, 2004b), combined with analysis of more reducible units of traits, goals, defenses, coping strategies, and so forth, generates the rich description of the human personality that defines the person-based approach. This scientific understanding of the person can form the basis for a person-based psychotherapy that places the complexity of human motive and meaning at the heart of the therapeutic work. Person-oriented therapists can indeed claim an intellectual and scientific justification for their commitment to taking the time to learn in depth about how an individual constructs an understanding of private thoughts and public encounters or employs narrative memories to guide and regulate moods and behaviors.

Finally, I propose that no single scientific method can capture the full complexity of the psychological person. We need to rely on psychometric measures, such as the Revised NEO Personality Inventory, (NEO PI-R); open-ended tasks such as the personal striving measure, narrative instruments such as the life-story interviews and self-defining memories, subjective interpretive analyses of relational therapy, and hermeneutic readings of the cultures in which the person is embedded to uncover the full range of human personality. Clearly, the breadth of this understanding is daunting, and many therapists would prefer to push forward while focusing on a partial aspect of the person or on one domain of the personality. Yet it is my conviction and perhaps my ideological assertion that the more we know about the person and the more means we use to accumulate this knowledge, the closer we can bring ourselves and our clients to a meaningful *and* ethical understanding of their lives. This understanding becomes a catalyst for personal change by deepening clients' insight into their own and others' motivations, by enabling them to weave together a coherent and purposeful narrative from their life story, and by empowering them to make more informed choices in their lives.

Of course, it is neither practical nor possible to bring all of these modes of knowing to bear on the work we do with our patients. They would be quickly out the door, looking for another therapist, while we continued our painstaking assessment of all these features. What I am arguing for is a sensibility that is open to this complexity and draws on it whenever possible. Certainly, there is time in the initial evaluation and interview to include some of the methods I have described in the previous chapters. Throughout the therapy, there are moments when further methods of data gathering and interpretation can be introduced. In the interest of learning about a particular domain of the person, self-report scales could be collected; strivings could be articulated; role-playing could be conducted; dreams and memories could be solicited and interpreted; poetry, music, and photography could be exchanged; spouses, partners, and family members could be brought into meetings to supply additional perspectives. Therapeutic efforts at understanding should have the same flexibility and breadth as the complicated and multilayered individuals who are the focus of that understanding. In their own way, both therapists and their clients need to embrace the poet Walt Whitman's invitation to uncover the souls of men and women,

> Undrape! you are not guilty to me, nor stale nor discarded,
> I see through the broadcloth and gingham whether or no,
> And am around, tenacious, acquisitive, tireless and cannot be
>   shaken away.
>   (1891–1892/1958, *Song of Myself,* Part 7, lines 21–24)

In this attitude of exploration, persons in therapy are most likely to feel free to examine the meanings and possibilities of who they are and who they might become. And at the very least, therapists protect themselves from a nonreflective embrace of treatment approaches that are inherently reductive and dismissive of individuals' complexity and depth. It was this spirit of openness and my unwillingness to pigeonhole that created the bridge to my businesswoman client whose story I told early in this chapter.

Ed Burke, a wise and beloved supervisor for my clinical training at the University of California–San Francisco, once expressed to me that therapy at its heart is nothing more than the ongoing effort to clarify our understanding of the people who have chosen to see us in treatment. Our dogged and comprehensive attempt to understand their world—its portions of suffering and solace—is where healing takes place. As individuals work with us to explain themselves, their own self-understanding deepens along with our awareness of who they are. Their insight and our expanding empathy combine to yield a rich and nurturing soil for growth and change.

This view, then, is ultimately the person-based perspective. It builds from the "humility" that was Allport's watchword. A person is extraordinarily intricate and difficult to know, and only the arrogant start from a premise of certainty in their presumed knowledge of another. In contrast, person-based therapists proceed with all due caution toward the understanding of another person and recruit all conceivable methods at their disposal. Their work is an ongoing project to be approached with curiosity and patience. Their yield is the opportunity to gain a brief glimpse into the life of another individual that reaffirms the wonder and grace of human life itself. In Chapter 7, I describe the application of this person-based approach in an actual case and also present research evidence that supports the value of this perspective.

7

Case Study of a
Person-Based Therapy

For the patient psychotherapists who have made their way through the preceding chapters on theory and research, it is time to explore the direct application of a person-based psychology to therapeutic practice. Drawing on an actual couples therapy from my clinical practice, I describe my work with Doug and Karen as they explore how to rebuild intimacy in their marriage of 25 years. (Each member of the couple gave informed consent to present their therapy and life stories on the condition of anonymity and the alteration of identifying details.) Since this book is focused on the individual person, I try to offer more individualized pictures of Doug and Karen than I might usually emphasize in my work with couples. In describing their couples work and how I have assisted their process of growth and change, I continue to use the three-domain framework and its relational context as the foundation of my person-based approach. This person-based therapy uses the same measures of traits, personal strivings, and self-defining memories that have been described in previous chapters. However, the benefit of couples therapy is that I can compare both individuals' self-assessments to the ways that their partners perceive them. It should be clear that these methods are applicable in either individual or couples treatment, but for my purpose here of explicating the relational dynamics of a person-based approach, the information available through couples work is invaluable.

BACKGROUND OF DOUG AND KAREN

Doug and Karen, now in their mid-40s, met shortly after finishing high school. After Karen became pregnant, they decided to marry and set up their own home. In time, they had two children, one daughter and one son. The daughter has now finished college and moved away, but their son is finishing high school and continues to live at home. Doug is the Director of Product Development for a medium-size information services company. Karen is a well-established investment broker for a major brokerage firm. Given that when they left home, both were working at a local retail store while attending college part-time, their career success and mutual level of accomplishment is nothing short of remarkable. Each of them presents as highly intelligent, attractive, and very likeable.

Doug comes from a large Greek family in which his father clearly ruled the roost and established his dominance over Doug's mother and the children. Doug was the oldest son, and his streak of independence often created sparks with his authoritarian father. Despite their disputes, Doug has always admired his father's success in the real estate business and the material comfort he gave to his family. When he struck out on his own with Karen, Doug was determined to remain independent of his father and to demonstrate that he too could become a financial success. Doug recalls his family as highly social and very close; there were many family gatherings, parties, and celebrations.

Karen was the product of a military romance between an American G. I. and a German shop girl in post-World War II Berlin. The couple moved back to the United States and had five more children, a mix of sons and daughters. Karen was brought up in a family that was much more reserved than Doug's. She was extremely shy when growing up and enjoyed the organized and structured home life provided by her parents. Not nearly as well off as Doug's family, Karen's family also had its share of serious illness, and one brother died at a young age of complications due to a rare blood disease.

Once Doug and Karen married in their late teens, they quickly settled into a routine of doing everything possible to build financial security for their young family. Doug never worked less than two jobs at a time and always managed to fit college courses into this demanding routine. Karen initially stayed at home to watch the baby but also picked up part-time work and college credits over the years of raising the two children. Doug's facility with computers allowed him to make several rapid career advances for someone of his youth and relative lack of educational credentials. Before long, he had caught the wave of the high-tech boom and gained even greater opportunities and financial prospects. At all times, he worked 70- to 80-hour weeks and continued his schooling.

As his successes accumulated, Karen slowly finished her business studies, then took a job with an investment brokerage firm. After starting with administrative duties, she gradually moved into the brokerage end, and in the last 10 years has made great strides in building a highly lucrative career.

In the previous 5 years, several converging events have caused Doug and Karen to look seriously at the quality of their marriage and even come to the point of questioning its continued viability. Perhaps the initial warning sign was when their adolescent son began to express extreme depression and a marked decline in school performance. His condition worsened to such an extent that he required multiple hospitalizations due to suicidal thoughts and threats. During this period of 2 years, Doug and Karen intermittently attended family therapy sessions, and at least one therapist called their attention to their son's perception of their frequent hostile exchanges and distance from each other. He had commented on how Doug seemed "absent" from the home and Karen always seemed be "nagging" her husband.

Terrified by their son's emotional struggles, Doug and Karen realized that they needed to scrutinize their own behavior in the family. Doug came to the conclusion that he had better slow down at work and in truth had reached a place where he could still be very successful without working quite as hard. Karen looked at her own efforts to manage everyone's life and keep the household afloat, while simultaneously building her career. She realized that to continue on this path would lead her to burnout, with the result of pleasing no one, including herself. At the same time, her brother's death as a young adult had cast a deep shadow over her life, pushing her to reconsider its pace and trajectory. She recognized that she needed to have more spiritual and life-affirming activities to regain a sense of harmony and balance.

As their son stabilized, and with their daughter off at college, Doug and Karen also realized that their shifting priorities had given them, perhaps for the first time in more than two decades, an opportunity to pursue their relationship with each other. Their success and the autonomy of their careers had afforded them (at least in theory) more possibilities than the typical couple for time together throughout the week and during the weekends. Ironically, this freedom to find each other had precipitated an escalation of tension and frustration beyond any level that they had previously reached in their marriage. Their repetitive fights centered on Karen's feeling that Doug did not respect her and did not truly care to spend time with her. In turn, Doug felt that Karen was constantly criticizing him and trying to control all facets of his life. Karen responded that Doug would probably prefer to have the kind of relationship that his father had with his mother in which he called all the shots and she accepted his will. After these arguments, Doug would slip out of the house and spend innumerable hours with friends, working on his sailboat or sports car—activities that seldom included Karen. When Doug was home, he often turned to watching sports on the large-screen television or surfing the Net on his computer. Meanwhile, Karen filled her life with her own activities—visiting with her family, jogging, and spending time with her friends. Their intimate life had grown increasingly sporadic and distant.

In a frank assessment of their goals for therapy, it became clear that they both still cared deeply for each other and did not want to sever their relationship. However, they realized that something fundamental had to change, since they were growing more and more angry and resentful toward each other. They agreed to commit to an initial series of 12 couples sessions that would entail learning more about their marriage, improving their communication, and building a more intimate and healthy relationship.

THE PERSON-BASED APPROACH:
LEARNING TO SEE THE OTHER PERSON AND ONESELF

In working with couples in conflict, I always suggest that one of the fundamental problems in their relationship is that they do not know each other well. This remark often brings incredulous and dismissive responses—"We know each other too well!! She doesn't have to finish her sentence and I know what she is going to say." I respond by saying, "This is exactly the problem—each of you *assumes* that you know your spouse almost as well as you know yourself. But what you may actually know is the stereotypes that you have created of each other." I explain how these caricatures of each other develop as a result of no longer fully listening to and looking at who one's partner really is. Much of couples work is about learning to *unlearn* these assumptions and taking the time to see one's partner with more observant eyes and to listen with more attuned ears, so that each person can capture the nuances and complexities of the other person that have been systematically overlooked. As each person sees the other more clearly, his or her own self-perception inevitably becomes more honest and insightful. Out of this self-scrutiny a more understanding and accepting relationship can emerge.

Step 1—NEO PI-R Self-Ratings

To begin this process of learning about each other and themselves, I asked Doug and Karen to fill out self-ratings on the NEO PI-R (see

Chapter 2) and then to rate each other on the same items. They were to fill out these questionnaires separately and return them to me; I then scored the questionnaires and shared the results with them both. Figure 7.1 shows the results for Doug self-ratings.

Doug's five domain scores reflected an overall pattern of positive adjustment with a low/very low score in Neuroticism and a high score in Extraversion. His Neuroticism score indicated his emotional stability, capacity to relax, and ability to handle stress. His high Extraversion score emphasized his strong positive energy, interpersonal warmth, and interest in challenging or exciting activities. He was average in Agreeableness and Conscientiousness, which indicates that he saw himself as reasonably conciliatory and trusting in his interactions and rather typical in his degree of dutifulness, organization, and achievement orientation. He was just below average in Openness, suggesting that he was a bit less flexible and slightly more conservative than the average person. In making these generalizations about these last three dimensions (O, A, C), one needs to be cautious, however, given the degree of scatter among the individual facets in each dimension. In fact, the average scores are, in part, a function of some high and low facets canceling each other out. In such cases, a facet analysis of each dimension may be more revealing than the overall scores.

Starting with Neuroticism, we see that Doug was very low in Anxiety and Self-Consciousness. This combination suggests a strong sense of confidence and calm, particularly when confronted with performance demands and social interactions. Given his status as corporate executive, this self-assurance and stability would certainly be an asset in his work. Similarly, he viewed himself as low, bordering on very low, in Depression and Vulnerability to Stress. Compared to these low and very low scores on the more reactive negative emotions (i.e., anxiety, depression, self-consciousness, and vulnerability to stress), he saw himself in the high average range on Anger/Hostility and in the high domain of Impulsiveness. This contrast points to Doug's willingness to acknowledge that there might be moments where he would be slightly more volatile and expressive of negative feelings than the average person. He also saw himself as much more inclined to give in to cravings or urges than the typical individual. Given his proneness to put on weight and some hard drinking in his earlier days, this self-assessment made sense.

Four of Doug's Extraversion facets were very high or high, and all of these elevated facets shared a common link to positive emotion, activity, and sensation-seeking. This tight cluster conveyed a strong desire for stimulation and fun, and an aversion to sitting still and passive pursuits. In contrast, the two scores that reflect the interpersonal aspect of Extraversion (Warmth and Gregariousness) were in the average and low

186

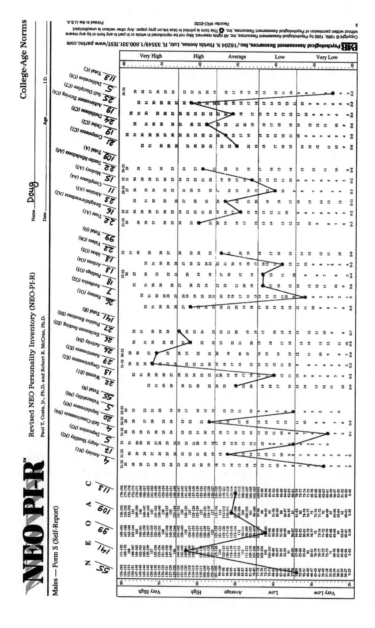

FIGURE 7.1. Doug's self-assessment. Profile form reproduced by special permission of the Publisher, Psychological Assessment Resources, Inc., 16204 North Florida Avenue, Lutz, Florida 33549, from the Revised NEO Personality Inventory by Paul T. Costa, Jr., PhD, and Robert R. McRae, PhD. Copyright 1978, 1985, 1989, 1992 by PAR, Inc. Further reproduction is prohibited without permission from PAR, Inc.

range, which means that his high E score was really due more to his strong activity orientation and less to his sociability.

Doug's lowest two Openness facets were in Aesthetics and Ideas, indicating a lack of interest or involvement in more artistic or philosophical pursuits. Combined with his low score in Feelings, these three facets coalesced around the picture of someone who is practical, action-oriented, and not prone to introspection or self-analysis of either thoughts or feelings. His low score in Actions conveyed an inclination to stick to his familiar routines and patterns of behavior with little inclination to break out of his preferred lifestyle. His two highest scores were an average level of Values (indicating a reasonable openness to other political, philosophical, or religious viewpoints) and a high score on Fantasy. In contrast to his marked lack of openness to exploring feelings and intellectual/artistic concerns, his high Fantasy score might be attributed to the creative entrepreneurial state of mind that had contributed to his career success. Throughout his life Doug had always been able to imagine the next three steps in his ascension up the corporate ladder. Similarly, much of his success had emerged from his ability to generate innovative and unexpected software solutions to challenging technological problems. With his thoughts preoccupied by technical problems and business schemes, it is no wonder that the other facets related to psychological introspection and awareness were at the opposite pole of this dimension.

Doug's two lowest Agreeableness facets were Compliance (low) and Modesty (low average). These scores fit well with an emerging pattern of someone who is self-confident and likely to stick to his own point of view despite the contrasting views of others. They also captured his competitive nature, which could border on aggressive at times. However, to complement these strong-willed qualities, his high scores in Trust and Tender-Mindedness highlighted an equal or greater capacity for compassion and concern for the suffering of others. They also reinforced his generally optimistic perspective and belief in the goodness of people. The contrast of his Agreeableness facets suggested the kind of person who forms intensely loyal friendships with a smaller circle of friends, but is unlikely to give up his values or preferences simply for the sake of ingratiating himself with others.

Finally, his Conscientiousness profile revealed high scores in Dutifulness and Self-Discipline, which should be no surprise given his remarkable history of hard work and commitment to supporting his family. The most striking score in this dimension was his extremely low score in Deliberation (his lowest score of all facets across all dimensions). This score reflected a marked tendency to make quick decisions and to throw caution aside. When combined with his high Impulsiveness scores and his strong Excitement-Seeking, we see a consistent profile of an individual who is action-oriented, risk-taking, and willing to act on "gut instinct." These characteristics certainly parallel the kind of entrepreneurial and aggressive business career in which Doug has thrived.

In considering patterns across dimensions and facets, we might emphasize Doug's high E and low N as an indicator of his stability, optimism, and overall general positive mental health. His low N and O point to his hyposensitivity to internal states, and his high E and low O indicate a kind of mainstream conventionality (to explore these patterns further, one can locate Doug on the Personality Styles graphs we used with Jennifer; see Chapter 2, Figure 2.3). His scores on facets related to activity, impulsivity, and challenge may be paired with his decreased scores on facets related to worry and concern, as well as philosophical or aesthetic rumination. The overall combination suggests a man of action who is not inclined to introspection about more emotional or relational issues. As Doug himself liked to put it, "I like to keep my focus on *transactions*—getting things done at work or around the house. It's not easy for me to sit still. Even if I have a game on, I will be looking at my computer, checking stock quotes, and leafing through a magazine at the same time."

Figure 7.2 presents Karen's NEO PI-R self-ratings. Her overall dimensions showed high scores in Openness, Agreeableness and Conscientiousness, an average score in Extraversion, and a very low score in Neuroticism. Her high Openness indicated sensitivity to inner feelings, intellectual curiosity, and a willingness to explore novel ideas or unconventional values. Her Agreeableness score reflected a high degree of compassion and concern for the feelings of others. Her high Conscientiousness pointed to a strong work ethic and moral code. Her very low Neuroticism suggested an absence of negative emotion and an impressive emotional stability.

Turning to a facet analysis, Karen was low or very low in all her Neuroticism facets, except Anxiety, which was low average. The combination of these facet scores conveyed the picture of someone who is extremely self-controlled and poised, even in the face of stress or challenge. In contrast to Doug's high score on Impulsiveness, Karen, saw herself as able to resist temptations and in very good control of her appetites and urges.

Her Extraversion facets were all clustered in the Average range with the exception of Excitement Seeking, which was very low. Once again, this disinclination to sensation-seeking and excitement was in marked contrast to Doug's penchant for high risk activity and challenge.

Karen's Openness facets fell in the average and high range. Her three high facets were Actions, Ideas, and Values, with Fantasy border-

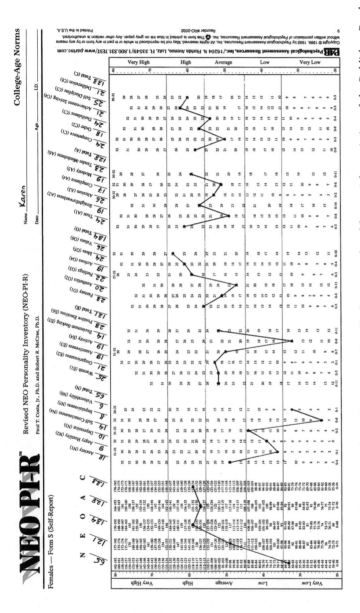

FIGURE 7.2. Karen's self-assessment. Doug's self-assessment. Profile form reproduced by special permission of the Publisher, Psychological Assessment Resources, Inc., 16204 North Florida Avenue, Lutz, Florida 33549, from the Revised NEO Personality Inventory by Paul T. Costa, Jr, PhD, and Robert R. McRae, PhD. Copyright 1978, 1985, 1989, 1992 by PAR, Inc. Further reproduction is prohibited without permission from PAR, Inc.

ing on high. This cluster pointed to her willingness to explore unconventional ways of thinking and being. It also reflected receptivity to philosophical and spiritual exploration, as well as alternative styles of life. In general, these results suggested a more flexible and introspective nature than what was revealed in Doug's profile.

Karen's Agreeableness facets hovered around the average and high range with higher scores in Trust, Altruism, and Tender-Mindedness. This trio suggested an idealistic and highly compassionate individual with a strong empathy for others' struggles and needs.

Finally, Karen's Conscientiousness facets were clustered closely together in the high (four facets) and average range (two facets). This profile conveyed a hard-working, competent individual with a clear moral purpose. Karen's two highest facets were Self-Discipline and Deliberation. Once again, her elevated score on Deliberation was the opposite of Doug's extremely low score on the same facet.

In looking at dimensional combinations, Karen's elevated Extraversion and very low Neuroticism pointed to her overall health and adjustment. Other combinations of her high Openness, Agreeableness, and Conscientious with her Low Neuroticism characterized her as a creative, innovated, upbeat, and easy-going person who is willing to explore her emotions, intellect, and spirituality. Combined with her strong scores in Trust, Altruism, and Tender-Mindedness, she did indeed fit her own self-description of a person guided by compassion and spiritual faith.

If I had only these self-assessments for Doug and Karen, I would certainly have a rich picture of who they were and how their relationship dynamics were likely to unfold. Both had strong commitments to different patterns of thought and action, but both were also very likely to assert the value of their respective positions. Doug might be likely to be restless in face-to-face conversation and uncomfortable with probing his feelings or private thoughts. He might want Karen to "get up and go with him"—to take on new activities or explore new challenges. Karen, on the other hand, might want Doug to spend more time with her in thoughtful conversations or simply share uncomplicated relaxing time together.

So far, these self-assessments simply reinforced Doug and Karen's time-hardened understanding of who they were. They carried around these self-images and projected them out to each other. The result was that they often ended up stuck in the same repetitive conflict with Karen wanting more personal "quality time" and Doug, resisting and resenting this pull on him that devalued his hobbies, sports, and time with friends. The next step in breaking down these familiar and comfortable positions within the couple was to examine their ratings of each other.

Step 2—Partners' Ratings of Each Other

A critical component of a person-based perspective is the recognition of our embeddedness in relationships with other important persons in our lives. We know ourselves through how others see us and ultimately we exist in the interstices of our own and others' perceptions of ourselves. Doug and Karen's ratings of each other added a critical additional layer to their and my understanding of the couple and their relationship dynamics. Figure 7.3 depicts Doug's ratings of himself in a serrated line and Karen's ratings of him in the solid line. Figure 7.4 depicts Karen's ratings of herself in the serrated line and Doug's ratings of her in the solid line. (Please note that while the numerical values for their self-ratings remain the same, the placement of their self-ratings on the Form R—Rater's Sheet changes due to different norms for observers' ratings versus self-ratings).

Clearly, Karen saw Doug as much higher on Neuroticism than he saw himself and as somewhat lower on Agreeableness. Doug's ratings of Karen were even more discrepant and negatively skewed than her ratings of him. He saw her as higher in Neuroticism and lower in Extraversion, Openness, and Agreeableness. He did see her as higher in Conscientiousness, but some of these ratings may have reflected his negative feelings about her overconcern for details and control. Looking at the Neuroticism facets, we see that he perceived her as more anxious, angry, and depressed, as well as more despairing, than she saw herself. With regard to Extraversion, he saw her as much less warm and friendly and more assertive than she saw herself. Doug also strongly rated Karen as lacking in an active, excitement-seeking, and positive approach to life. On all dimensions of Openness (except the Feeling facet, which may have reflected his perception that she was "too sensitive"), Doug saw Karen as much more closed and rigid than she saw herself. On the Agreeableness dimension, similar to Karen's perceptions of him, Doug saw her as less trusting, altruistic, modest, conciliatory, and tender than she perceived herself. Finally, he did appear to rate Karen's competence, ambition, moral strength, self-discipline, and self-control even higher than she had rated herself.

Given that in their professional positions they both relied heavily on data interpretation, Doug and Karen took the results of the NEO PI-R very seriously. As Doug put it, "There it is, right on the test; we can't deny there is a giant gap between us." Karen agreed, but stated that she was a bit shaken by the depth of Doug's negative picture of her. She certainly did not want to be perceived as the kind of person he had described with his ratings. It was not at all how she felt about herself, but she could indeed see how their conflicts had led Doug to construe her in

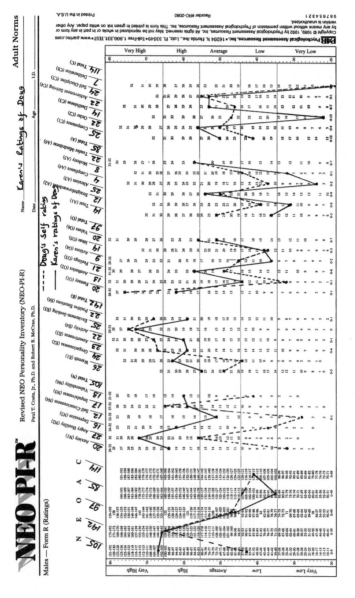

FIGURE 7.3. Karen's ratings of Doug. Doug's self-assessment. Profile form reproduced by special permission of the Publisher, Psychological Assessment Resources, Inc., 16204 North Florida Avenue, Lutz, Florida 33549, from the Revised NEO Personality Inventory by Paul T. Costa, Jr., PhD, and Robert R. McRae, PhD. Copyright 1978, 1985, 1989, 1992 by PAR, Inc. Further reproduction is prohibited without permission from PAR, Inc.

192

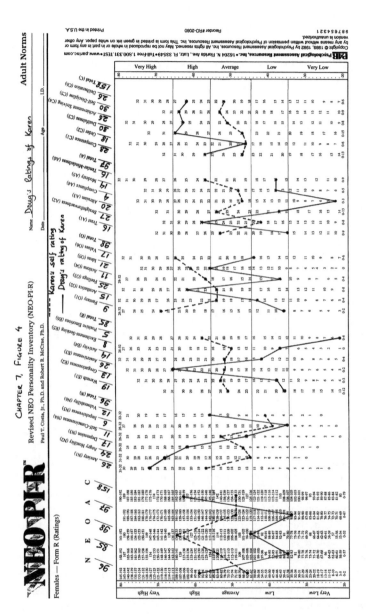

FIGURE 7.4. Doug's ratings of Karen. Doug's self-assessment. Profile form reproduced by special permission of the Publisher, Psychological Assessment Resources, Inc., 16204 North Florida Avenue, Lutz, Florida 33549, from the Revised NEO Personality Inventory by Paul T. Costa, Jr., PhD, and Robert R. McRae, PhD. Copyright 1978, 1985, 1989, 1992 by PAR, Inc. Further reproduction is prohibited without permission from PAR, Inc.

193

this way. Doug conceded that he might not be fully acknowledging how sad and frustrated he had been about the quality of their relationship; the results indicated to him that they did indeed need some help and had to do some work to change these destructive views of each other.

Shortly after this assessment, Karen had to undergo an extensive medical procedure, and then I was out of the country on a sabbatical leave. It was several months before we resumed our work together, but there had been little change in Doug and Karen's relationship dynamics. When they returned to treatment and began regular weekly sessions, they were still engaging in frequent arguments at home and tended to avoid focused time with each other that was not shared with family or friends. Karen expressed her strong feeling that this situation was no longer acceptable to her; they had to take steps to improve their relationship or else take seriously the idea of separating.

Drawing on some of the fundamental techniques of couples work, nicely described by Hendrix (1988), I asked Doug and Karen if they were willing to agree to commit to the relationship for the next 3 months and to at least 12 sessions of meeting with me. With this commitment from both of them, I then told them that the NEO PI-R had demonstrated how much they still needed to learn (or unlearn) about each other. In the interest of helping them learn about each other, I first needed to know how they scheduled their time and the nature of their interactions with each other. Each member of the couple created for me a detailed schedule of how each day of a typical week and weekend proceeded. We looked closely at how their time was allotted and when they came together to share time with each other. We also looked at how time was divided among work, household duties, and leisure.

Their schedules revealed how separate their lives had become over their long marriage despite the fact that they were often in their home together. After long hours of work, on some nights, they would come together for meals, but on other nights grab food on the run while continuing to work late at home or go out for exercise or contact with friends. When Doug and Karen did eat together, they would then migrate to separate parts of the house, engaging in their own private activities (Doug watching sports or surfing the Net; Karen reading or watching television; activities that Hendrix calls "exits"). On weekends, Doug would often spend long days and some evenings with his friends, sailing or playing tennis, followed by time at his club. They rarely planned a date with each other or created an occasion that emphasized their sense of romance or of being a couple. Other social time was taken up with family visits on both sides.

As we reviewed all of this information, I began to talk with them about the concept of "I" versus "we." Much of their life seemed to focus on "contractual" agreements made between two separate parties. They would talk about what "I like to do" and what the partner "likes to do." They saw their activities as often taking place in spite of or with the permission of the partner. There was very little sense of shared time, of how "we like to be together" or what "we would like to do as a couple." In fact, it often seemed that the idea of thinking about what was "best for them as a couple" was a foreign concept. They were much more comfortable thinking about what was best for each individual in the relationship and would then set about negotiating when interests came into conflict. I pointed out that the core of my approach to couples work was to encourage them to see themselves as two persons *embedded in a relationship* and that they needed to make a constant return to the simple question of what was best for this relationship. For their marriage to move forward, they needed to shift fundamentally from "me" thinking to "we" thinking. I pointed out that the NEO PI-R ratings had demonstrated to them that they did not exist in isolation: Their personalities were interactions of their own self-perceptions and the perceptions that others held of them.

Building on these ideas, we were able to examine how the most basic structural work of examining their schedules could reveal long-standing and obsolete conceptions of each other. For example, despite the fact that Karen was now a highly paid professional with a full-time job, she was still responsible for all weekend housework and shopping. This imbalance in the home was a vestige of the original arrangement of their marriage and of Doug's experience during his own upbringing. After exploration of the harm that this continued role for Karen was doing to their relationship dynamic, they agreed to hire some help. However, what emerged in their efforts to hire someone was a continued struggle over how active a role Doug might play in this task and whether Karen could relinquish control in letting Doug pursue this responsibility. Was there a way that they could make this change by viewing this goal in the context of connection to each other rather than as a concession of one person to another? Ultimately, they tentatively developed a way of working together to find someone. The subsequent success of this decision (with the reduction of workload for Karen) became an important symbol of their new, mutual efforts to find solutions for improving the relationship.

However, as the weeks continued, the challenge of actually getting to know each other and spending dedicated time with each other became more apparent. Doug continued to resent Karen's perceived "demands" on his time, and Karen also persisted in feeling that Doug was not really interested in her or respectful of her as a person or companion. She felt that he was sometimes dismissive of her wishes and that he occasionally put her down in front of their friends.

This tension can be best exemplified by an incident that took place during their annual winter trip, which happened to be on a tropical cruise. They were making a genuine effort to share time together and were even enjoying much more intimacy than usual. However, Doug insisted on smoking cigars on two of the five nights they were on the trip. Karen detested the smell, even though he smoked them outside the cabin and away from her. The rest of the night she felt repelled from any closeness with Doug. His refusal to give up the cigars and her intolerance of them led to several tense moments on the trip and a bitter aftertaste regarding their experience together. As I discussed all the implications of this dispute with them, Doug recognized that being so close with Karen night after night stirred up many powerful feelings within and left him feeling a need to withdraw from this intense intimacy; the cigar provided a convenient vehicle to make an "exit" from the relationship (this situation demonstrated the opposite of Freud's valuable dictum that "sometimes a cigar is only a cigar"). Karen was aware that her concern for control might have led Doug to feel that he indeed needed some air away from her.

Returning to the theme of a person-based therapy, it was becoming clear in the couples work that creating time together or urging more joint activities were effective strategies up to a point, but that a true movement from "me to we" would require a deepening understanding of who each person was in the relationship, and what goals and defenses each contributed to the ongoing couples dynamic. To get at these questions, we moved next to the second domain of the person—Characteristic Adaptations—and each person's personal strivings.

EXAMINING DOUG'S AND
KAREN'S PERSONAL STRIVINGS

I asked Doug and Karen each to perform the homework assignment of generating a list of 10 personal strivings (see Chapter 3 for more details on this method), using the standard "I typically try to . . . " stem. I stipulated that they could not share their list with each other until we met in the next session. Doug's list is displayed in Table 7.1 and Karen's in Table 7.2. Before Doug shared his list, I asked Karen to imagine what would be on his list. Karen's vision of Doug's strivings appears in Table 7.3. Doug's vision of Karen's strivings appears in Table 7.4.

Looking at Doug's list first, we see powerful evidence for his status as "the transactional man." His list was filled with concrete actions and contained not a single reference to an emotional state or introspective activity. He clearly divided up his strivings into domains of discrete

TABLE 7.1. Doug's Personal Strivings

1. Plan my work week in advance.
2. Make certain that the financials are in good order.
3. Exercise.
4. Stay in contact with kids.
5. Make certain that the "household" paperwork is organized.
6. Stay "in touch" with news and current events/read as much as possible.
7. Spend time with Karen.
8. Keep ahead of my workload.
9. Talk to my friends.

tasks, and his approach reflected his extreme responsibility, highlighting terms such as *plan, make certain, stay in contact, stay in touch,* and *keep ahead.* His children are fourth on his list; his parents are sixth; Karen is seventh; and his friends are ninth (he claimed that he could not come up with a tenth striving). With regard to his striving scores for agency and communion, Doug showed a clear balance between these two motives, with four strivings that were communal and five that were more agentic and achievement-based.

Turning to Karen's vision of Doug's ratings, we should note that she saw Doug as strongly oriented toward family and friends, as well as his work and leisure activities. She placed "Do well" as his top goal, suggesting that she perceived his success and competitive orientation as ma-

TABLE 7.2. Karen's Personal Strivings

1. Be optimistic and hopeful—have faith.
2. Understand others' points of view.
3. Talk to my family.
4. Find laughter, quiet, calmness.
5. Take care of myself and people around me.
6. Tell my family I love them and care.
7. Work hard at everything I try.
8. Think of ways to spend more time with Doug (do his sports, try things he likes, etc.).
9. Think people are good.
10. Balance work and family.
11. Think before I speak and when I speak.
12. Be sincere.

TABLE 7.3. Karen's Vision of Doug's Personal Strivings

1. Do well.
2. Spend time with family.
3. Spend time with friends.
4. Have fun.
5. Work hard.
6. Make time to do the things he enjoys.
7. Try to contact and connect with the kids.
8. Help out around the house.
9. Think of Karen.

jor driving forces in his life. In contrast, she put "Think about Karen" at the last of his nine strivings, which, given its location of seventh place on his actual list, was not a bad assessment of where he placed the priority of their relationship at that time.

Karen's striving list stood in marked contrast to Doug's approach to my request. Whereas he was one striving short, she provided two extra strivings. If Doug's list lacked emotional and introspective terms, Karen's list was replete with these kinds of concerns. Her list included multiple references to *thinking* and *being*, as well as trying to *understand* others. She mentioned *hope, faith, laughter, calm, love,* and *sincerity*—all aspects of her inner life, as opposed to the external world of transactions. Four of her first six strivings involved the care of and connection to other people, especially her family. Similar to Doug, Karen placed a direct mention of time with her spouse rather low on her list—the eighth of 12 strivings. Also, similar to Doug, Karen displayed a mixture of communal and agentic strivings, with her emphasis decidedly on the communal side. Repeating her openness to philosophical and spiritual concerns that emerged on the NEO PI-R, she placed having faith at the

TABLE 7.4. Doug's Vision of Karen's Personal Strivings

1. Typically be in close contact with kids.
2. Typically make time for us.
3. Manage the household.
4. Stay ahead of her work.
5. Find time to relax.
6. Like to be right.
7. Like to make her voice heard.

very top of her list. In accordance with her high Agreeableness ratings on the NEO PI-R, Karen's strivings indicated that she tried very hard to trust in others and to accommodate herself to their points of view.

Doug's vision of Karen's strivings made a clear point of emphasizing that she placed her priorities on family and her relationship with him. He also displayed a respect for her efforts to manage home and work. However, he could not resist using the exercise to make a jibe at Karen about her efforts to assert herself and "be right." What seemed strongly missing from his vision of her most important goals was Karen's investment in her own and others' emotional worlds. This omission on Doug's part could easily lead to a perception that Karen's efforts to share time with him were in the interest of control rather than an intense desire for connection and intimacy.

After they had shared their respective lists and discussed the discrepancies in their visions of each other, we saw again how their combined lists reflected the complementary nature of their relationship. Doug was an effective manager of their external world—the universe of work, finances, and household maintenance. Karen contributed in these areas but assigned herself the primary role of managing the interior world of the couple—as caretaker of the emotions and particular needs of each member of the family. In recognizing the weight of each of their responsibilities, I asked Doug and Karen not only to acknowledge with gratitude what each was accomplishing for the family but also to consider how they could ease each other's burdens. In particular, I encouraged them to work a bit harder at learning to adopt a bit of their partner's style. For Doug, this meant making more effort to check in with Karen and to take the time to communicate his feelings to her. For Karen, greater balance would require her to be a bit more patient with his transactional and parallel style of being together. In such moments, she might have to resist pressuring Doug for a sense of connection or affirmation. Both indicated a willingness to try these shifts in their usual patterns, assuming that each partner recognized and rewarded the other's efforts. They left this session feeling once again that they had learned to see their partner in a slightly different light, a vantage point that promoted a better sense of trust and a reduction in hostile attributions.

Simultaneous with these person-based exercises, I also worked closely with Karen and Doug on improving their style of communication with each other. I emphasized that the key form of learning about each other was to ask questions and make sure that they understood fully the answers that they received. I made them practice restatements of each other's replies, along with demonstrating a commitment to "I feel" statements and a rejection of "mind reading" and assumptions (e.g., "When you assume, you make an ass out of you and me"). Their level of comfort with each other slowly increased, and the reduction in hostility and arguments was also notable. They planned more time together and recognized that careful communication about each other's whereabouts and activity plans went a long way in reducing their tension and frustration with each other.

Yet despite this considerable progress, they were still likely to get into small snits over Karen's requests for Doug's time and his sense that she was too controlling of his social activities. In turn, she felt that Doug often undid the benefit of some of their times together by subsequently forgetting to check in or by scheduling an event with a friend or one of his relatives without consulting their mutual calendar. We called these "cigar moments"—instances in which Doug seemed to pull back from their increased intimacy. In order to get at these inured patterns, it was necessary that I move the therapy to still another level of analysis and mutual understanding that captured the way their life histories seemed to interfere with their efforts at building a better relationship in the present. In reference to examining their histories, I talked about the how every couples therapy has "ghosts" in the room—the traces of family interaction patterns that the partners had repeatedly observed as children in their families of origin. These early, learned patterns filled the spaces of the room with their spectral presences, haunting and trapping the couple in misunderstandings and misreadings of current efforts at healthier interaction. To exorcize these ghosts and neutralize their influence on the couple's relationship, I proposed another homework assignment—the recall of three self-defining memories that would convey to each other the most important themes and conflicts in their respective lives. Once again, I asked them not to share the memories with each other until they came to their next meeting with me.

KAREN'S AND DOUG'S SELF-DEFINING MEMORIES

Drawing on the instructions from the self-defining memory request (see Chapter 4), Doug and Karen had each identified three of the most significant memories from the past. Karen went first and described the three self-defining memories listed in Table 7.5. After she finished narrating each memory, I asked Karen to tell Doug what the memory meant to her and what themes from her life that it best seemed to capture. In recounting her first memory of being picked on at school, Karen emphasized her sense of being different—both because of her foreign background and her shyness. She explained that the memory was for her an example of how she is slow to trust people outside her most immediate circle. Her next memory only reinforced the theme of the centrality of family and

TABLE 7.5. Karen's Self-Defining Memories

1. I was picked on a lot in elementary school. It had to do with a few different things. I was not like other kids—my mom spoke very little English and I had a bit of an accent. Kids would call me Nazi or say things about Hitler. One day, waiting for the bus, this boy rolled a trash barrel at me and slammed my knee. It was all bloody and the school nurse cleaned it up for me, but it was like the show-and-tell all day.

This memory showed me that not all people are nice. People can be quick to judge. I felt hurt and confused, but I don't remember feeling angry.

2. I almost lost my father during Christmas when I was 8 years old. He fell 60 feet at a construction site, crushed both legs, and damaged his kidneys. I was terrified and everyone in my household was racing all around; there was crying and chaos. Our neighbors took us children and made Christmas for us. It took months, but he recovered.

I did see how much family and friends could pull together and I learned a lot about the importance of the people who are close to you.

3. All of the events around the diagnosis and loss of my brother at age 27. . . . It was from a rare blood disease. We were shocked and fearful, followed by overwhelming sadness. I saw again how much family can do—how we pulled together. It helped me through this time. There was such a void in my life. It brought me back to church. Throughout his whole illness, I kept asking: Why did this happen to him? I had no answers, but at the end there was an odd occurrence. It was like I reached another level of being. I saw that there was always hope, always something good. When he finally passed, he defied the doctor's predictions, lasted through the weekend when there appeared to be no chance. That night of his death, all at once, petals fell off a rose, the door flew open, a picture frame that belonged to him fell off the shelf, and wind was blowing so hard, I suddenly heard his voice, saying "I'm okay now."

I know people may think that I just imagined these events or they were coincidence, but I know that something larger than myself was communicating to us, that my brother was still reaching out to me, still trying to give comfort to our family.

close friends in her life. Nearly losing her father when she was so young filled Karen with a potent sense of the fragility of life. The kindness of her other family members and the neighbors showed Karen that the only antidote to these kinds of tragedies was to rely on comfort and support from people who know one best.

Finally, Karen's third memory took this progression from injury to life-threatening accident to its logical conclusion, the death of a loved one. For Karen, the death of her brother exceeded all pain that she could have previously imagined and threatened to drop her into a blackness that she might not ever have shaken. The redeeming moments of this traumatic loss were her brother's courage and a moment of spiritual connection, when her brother spoke to her after he had departed. Karen struggled for many months with an overwhelming sadness, bordering on total despair, but at each point of giving up, she found that her faith restored her sense of purpose and belief in the value of life, and the blessings that life had to offer.

Doug listened very attentively to Karen and indicated that the last two memories were ones that he might have predicted she would have chosen. He had not expected the first memory about her being picked on to play such a prominent role for her. He had not realized how different and isolated she had felt. I indicated that we would pick up further on his reactions later on, and asked that he continue with the exercise and present his memories.

Doug went on to describe his memories in less detail than Karen, but with a surprising degree of emotion (see Table 7.6). All three memories held a rather somber and painful aspect for him. Although his second memory, the birth of his first child, contained moments of elation

---

TABLE 7.6. Doug's Self-Defining Memories

1. My first memory is about the death of my cousin Tina, who was 22 and killed by a drunk driver. She was the daughter of my mother's brother and we grew up together. It was my first recognition that mortality was out there. I was in my early 20s and I couldn't cope. I wasn't ready for something like this. It had a big impact, seeing my aunt and uncle's pain. I was filled with rage at the driver, wanted to kill him.

I am not sure what I learned except that you can lose life at any moment. It's a memory of such pain that I also try to forget it at times.

2. I recall the birth of my first child. It was a huge sense of responsibility. It set the tone for the rest of our lives—drove me to be successful. I felt everyone was counting on me financially and for other support as well. It was also a happy event. I was filled with love just looking at her. But it forced decisions. We had her before we were married and we were both from religious families. There was a lot of stress. We married and moved into our own place. I took responsibility for all our affairs. We grew up fast, and this defined who we are. I think for this reason my first child has always been very special.

3. My last memory is of when my son received a diagnosis of major depression. It was outside my control and I couldn't fix it. I couldn't make it better on my own. I am not an emotional person. It pushed more emotion on me than I could even handle. I was distraught, suicidal. I went for a walk with my pistol and really thought about ending it. I was desperate and I was thinking that maybe my own death would cause him to see life as precious. I would have traded my own life for his in a heartbeat, if I felt it would have made a difference. I felt such guilt for his illness. Maybe I hadn't given him what he needed—been too hard on him or not shown enough affection. There was my arrogance that I could do anything—solve any problem, that I was a survivor, but his illness had me beat. I remember begging the hospital to take him after another episode of his hurting himself. I finally broke down in tears.

and love for him, Doug chose to emphasize the sense of responsibility it created in his life. He spoke about how he was determined to prove to his father that he could make it on his own and become every bit as successful. In talking about this memory, it was almost as if Doug could identify when the yoke of "provider" was laid upon his shoulders, a duty that he had not once put aside ever since. He managed to convey both the extraordinary pride and the burden that were simultaneously transferred to his person at that moment of her birth.

With the stories of their memories recounted, I asked Doug and Karen to reflect on common themes they had detected. Both noted the overall dark quality of their memories—that each had chosen to highlight traumatic or painful episodes in their lives. I mentioned that in my research this was not all that unusual; people do seem to learn more from moments of loss or conflict in their lives (cf. Thorne et al., 2004). However, notably, not one of the six memories conveyed an unquestioned sense of joy or triumph. They did indeed seem to be operating with a certain weight of sadness bearing down on their lives together.

I thought about the types of analysis that I could bring to understanding the memories. From a structural standpoint, two of Karen's memories were of very specific events described with imagery and detail (i.e., being hit by the trash barrel and the day of her brother's death); the third was more episodic, blending several days involving her father's injury and the aftermath. In contrast, Doug recalled two of his three memories in a summary fashion (i.e., his cousin's death and his daughter's birth), leaving out any specific imagery or details of the events. His tendency to stay at an abstract and general descriptive level only made the last memory's specific imagery of his nighttime walk with his pistol more compelling and raw. Doug's general memories in conjunction with his "transactional" strivings point to his overall inclination to avoid connecting to and expressing strong emotion. However, due to the work he had been doing in the couples therapy, and through the family counseling he had done over the years in support of his son, Doug was willing to take more of a risk and let some of his emotion come through in his last memory.

In thinking about the thematic qualities of their memories, although all of his memories involved interpersonal events, Doug tended to emphasize the agentic aspects of these experiences. In his memory of his cousin's death, he stressed the fact that he was not ready to recognize the concept of mortality—that he could not cope with the event, that he was not "ready." His daughter's birth led him to acknowledge his responsibility and commitment to succeed. Finally, his son's hospitalization for depression drove Doug to a sense of utter powerlessness, followed by the fantasy that if he killed himself, he might be able to influence his son's willingness to embrace life. All three memories were linked by Doug's concern about agentic competence and his image of being in control over the vagaries of life.

In contrast, Karen's memories were extraordinarily focused on communion and the threat to relationship. She depicted a potentially hostile world in which family offers the ultimate outpost of comfort and safety. In addition, connection to family and the love offered by family members provide a conduit to a spiritual communion that gives day-to-day life an overarching order and purpose. When McAdams (1988) codes the intimacy motive, one scoring criterion is the connection not simply to intimate others but to a transcendent element, whether it be nature or a higher spiritual being. Thematically, then, Doug's and Karen's memories captured the two very different stances that they could take in their relationship as a couple—one stance based in control of self and mastery of the surrounding world, and the other in letting the self find solace in others and through submission to a transcendent faith.

I had asked Karen and Doug to tell each other what they wanted their partner to learn from their memories. Karen had pointed out that she wanted Doug to know how important family was to her and how much time together mattered to her. She wanted him to know how skeptical she was about the goodness of people, and that this was why she placed so much stock in family and on the most intimate of relationships. Time with Doug and with her family took precedence over all other ways that Karen could spend time in her life. Her father's near-death and her brother's early death had taught her this lesson.

When Doug answered my question, I saw for the first time in the work we had done together a break in his controlled style. He said that he wanted Karen to know that though his emotions were not on the surface, his feelings were still there. As Doug tried to say this out loud, his voice caught slightly, and he seemed momentarily overcome. Karen said that she knew this, but that he tended to show his feelings more through anger. Doug mentioned that he had cried when his cousin died, but Karen pointed out that he had also put a hole through a wall out of rage.

I then asked what they had learned about each other that they had not known before. Karen said that the struggles in her own life had taught her about accepting things that cannot be controlled. She had never understood that Doug's nearly attempting suicide (which he had disclosed to her before) was in his mind an act to help *control* the situation. For the first time, she now realized that Doug's impulse to take his life was not born out of selfishness, guilt, or a desire to escape from the pain. She saw now that Doug saw his own death at that moment as an act of sacrifice— a willingness to give up himself if it could save his son. Karen saw more clearly and more persuasively than ever before that Doug's greatest struggle at that moment was not with death or pain or fear, but with the idea that he could not make a difference, that he could not have an influence over the way events transpired.

At this moment in the room, there was a palpable change in how Karen and Doug were with each other—a softening of their respective stances and a reduction in their distance. In that juncture, as I have described in an earlier chapter, "Love was in the air." The goal of a person-based approach in couples work (or in any form of therapy) is to help individuals see others and themselves with new eyes, to let go of older views and see the full complexity that defines our human nature. By allowing love to enter the room, they could look for convergences of understanding rather than the aspects of their persons that defined their differences and divergences. By focusing on the effort to understand each other more fully, they could seek ways to make the relationship the positive force that Karen believed to be the essence of her spiritual faith.

In the pattern of their relationship, this insight meant recognition by Karen that moments in which Doug felt a potential loss of control due to intimacy were likely to lead to a sense of alarm and withdrawal in him. In turn, this withdrawal provoked her anger and attributions about his lack of caring for her. Doug needed to understand that his use of exits would undermine the sense of connection that was of paramount importance to Karen. Karen, for her part, needed to let go of the notion that these exits were expressions of Doug's lack of affection for her.

When such moments occurred, it helped to recall the memories' images, similar to the "cigar moments" to which I referred earlier. The memories were indeed what Greenberg (2002) dubbed "emotional handles" for this pattern: They served as a metaphor to remind the couple of this familiar sequence in which Karen's striving for intimate connection would come into conflict with Doug's fear of loss of control. The solution was not to harden each other's respective position, but instead to recognize each other's needs and limitations, and then look for middle ground.

This notion of a nuanced and fluid understanding of how the couple could be with each other was a long way from the polarized visions of each other that Doug and Karen had initially provided on the NEO PI-R. It moved them from "me to we." They were indeed learning to fill in the full person for each other, to move beyond the initial generalizations that caught them up in an accusatory and self-defeating cycle. They were now starting to see themselves as part of a larger structure, a relational matrix that encompassed both of their individual personalities and melded them to a unique third entity—the relationship that they had created together.

The session ended with their agreement to renew their efforts to make time for each other and to seek ways to bring pleasure to each other's lives. Karen proposed that the happiness they achieved in their relationship could indeed be understood as a gift to those who had passed away and were now known only through memory. In order to make these commitments concrete, they again promised to share their schedules with each other and to make sure that their weekend would be organized around making time to spend with each other. Their goal was to show greater patience and trust in these preparations, while mutually acknowledging the other person's perspective.

Over the months that I continued to work with Doug and Karen, we were able to make repeated reference to the themes and images raised by the memories they recalled. They made genuine progress (with to-be-expected setbacks) in building a greater intimacy and reenergizing their relationship. They continued to practice the communication skills they had learned and to show both greater love and respect toward each other than they had at any prior point in their marriage. Perhaps most important, they continued to learn about each other, to remain open to the possibility that the person with whom they had shared more than 25 years *and* the relationship that they had built were still not fully known and still worth discovering.

CONCLUDING THOUGHTS: WHAT IS A PERSON?

In providing this example of person-based therapy, I do not at all propose that I am offering a new school of therapy or a set of practices that represent a radical departure from either traditional insight-oriented therapies or more contemporary cognitive-behaviorally informed therapies. Clearly, my practice of therapy incorporates valuable components of each of these perspectives. The difference lies in two fundamental issues, both of which incorporate my allegiance to a larger person-based psychology. First, I have demonstrated that my methods of assessment and intervention blend the instruments of academic personality research (e.g., the NEO PI-R, personal strivings assessment, life histories, and self-defining memories) with the interpretive orientation of relational psychodynamic therapy (e.g., as depicted in the work of Ogden, Mitchell, and others). Second, and again borrowing from personality psychology (as I have conceived its person-based format), I am committed to helping my clients pursue the fullest understanding of themselves possible, as opposed to a practice of therapy that is focused primarily on the treatment of symptoms and illnesses, or that necessarily subscribes to a reductive metapsychology of fundamental drives or impulses.

A person-based therapy also takes a stand about the nature of inquiry into the understanding of the person. It specifies the domains of investigation of the person that are drawn from McAdams's three domains of personality. It argues that we will learn much by studying individuals' overarching disposition (traits), characteristic adaptations (strivings, defenses, coping strategies, cognitive strategies, life tasks, etc.), and narrative identity (life histories, self-defining memories, scripts, personal myths, etc.). The combined knowledge provided by these three domains will go a long way toward providing a fuller picture of the individual than has heretofore been possible.

In conceptualizing a person-based approach to psychotherapy, I have demonstrated fruitful applications of all three domains to the treatment of a couple in marital distress. In recent years, there has been an explosion of interest in particular in the application of the third narrative domain to psychotherapy. Since the narrative domain is most centrally involved with the questions of meaning making and understanding that form the heart of a person-based perspective, I would like to take a bit more time in calling attention to these narrative applications to therapeutic work.

For example, James Pennebaker and his colleagues (Pennebaker, 1995, 1997; Pennebaker & Francis, 1996; Pennebaker & Seagal, 1999) have demonstrated that undisclosed traumas have the potential to detract from physical and mental health. In contrast, self-disclosure that allows for meaningful analysis and interpretation of traumatic events is conducive to better psychological and physical health, as well as to improvement in immune functioning (Pennebaker & Keough, 1999). According to Pennebaker and Keough, self-disclosure in narrative form enables individuals to reframe the meaning of traumatic experiences, to integrate these experiences into a sense of identity, and to remake newer, stronger selves in spite of past trauma.

Laura King, another researcher who studies narrative, has found that individuals who struggle to make sense of difficult transitions in their lives, as opposed to denying or simply applying "happy endings" to these transitions, show greater overall maturity and enhanced wisdom in their lives. For example, in one study of divorced women and another of parents of children with Down syndrome, she was able to find correlations between a greater willingness to tell narratives that incorporate loss and conflicted feelings and higher levels of ego development and maturity, both concurrently and longitudinally (King & Raspin, 2004; King et al., 2000).

Leslie Greenberg and his colleagues at the York Psychotherapy Research Center in Toronto have used single-case analyses to demonstrate the therapeutic efficacy of emotional differentiation and disclosure through the vehicle of narrative. Greenberg and Angus (2004) wrote:

The narrative organization of emotional experience—in which intentions, purposes, expectations, hopes, and desires are articulated—is
what allows us to reflexively understand what an experience means to
us and says about us. (p. 332)

Greenberg and Angus (1995, cited in Greenberg & Angus, 2004) provided an illustration from a psychotherapy transcript of a "good
outcome" psychotherapy. Working with the client in an "empty chair"
intervention, the therapist assisted the client in applying more subtle
metaphorical and emotionally differentiated language to her struggle
with negative feelings toward her husband. The client used narrative de-
vices to articulate that her husband was not simply unloving, but "steps
on her" and made her feel like a "slave" who did everything for him and
the children but never felt that they "do anything together" (pp. 340–
341). Greenberg and Angus demonstrated that these movements toward
more descriptive, metaphorical, and emotion-focused language were associated with greater insight, better outcomes, and more lasting change
in psychotherapy.

Just as meaning making and differentiation of emotion processes
can emerge from attention to the narratives that individuals form of the
events in their lives, so too can narratives in psychotherapy be studied
for what they reveal about relationship patterns. For over 25 years,
Luborsky and colleagues (Book, 1998, 2004; Crits-Christoph & Luborsky, 1998; Luborsky, 1997, 1998; Luborsky & Crits-Christoph, 1998)
have used narratives generated in psychotherapy to extract relationship
themes that present repetitive problems for individuals. These *core
conflictual relationship themes* (CCRTs) can be reliably coded from psychotherapy transcripts and tracked in the transference relationship with
the therapist, as well in significant relationships with partners, family
members, friends, and coworkers. The CCRT consists of a relationship
episode (RE), which is any account of an interaction with another person. Within a given RE, one can identify a wish (W), response from
other (RO), and response from self (RS). For example, in my work with
Doug and Karen, we might take the cigar episode as one incidence of an
RE. If we were to focus on Karen, we might describe her W for Intimacy
with Doug. Doug's RO is to offer intimacy initially but then withdraw
(by smoking the cigar) when he feels too vulnerable. In considering Karen's RS, we might note that Luborsky distinguishes between the behavioral RS and the affective RS. Behaviorally, Karen rejects intimacy with
Doug, while affectively she feels angry, hurt, and rejected.

The goals of CCRT therapy are to help clients identify these repetitive relationship patterns in their lives and then to explore how to
modify elements within the patterns that reduce self-defeating aspects.

Exploration of CCRTs can lead to modification of wishes, alternative interpretations of others' responses, and/or changes in one's own response. CCRT therapy can aid the client to achieve better communication with the other person about the dynamics and frustrations of the particular relationship pattern. As Crits-Christoph and Luborsky (1998) demonstrated, a decline in ROs and RSs over the course of therapy was correlated with a reduction in symptoms of distress and conflict. Interestingly, while the original ROs and RSs were reduced, the frequency of the initial W stayed constant, suggesting that more effective interpersonal strategies for achieving the desired state were being employed.

The CCRT method provides a perfect bridge between the importance of narrative to a concept of the person and the relational context in which that narrative is embedded. As Chapter 5 of this volume explored in great detail, a person-based psychology cannot treat the person as simply an independent entity built on the three domains of traits, characteristic adaptations, and narratives. Recognition of the inherently social nature of the human being requires that we expand our understanding of the person to include the relational matrix in which all human beings find themselves. We first emerge from another person's body; we live all our lives among other human beings (and if not literally, then with their voices and presences inside our thoughts), and our greatest fear is to die alone. The pervasive influence of other people on our lives is expressed not only in our immediate interpersonal relationships with family, partners, friends, neighbors, coworkers, teachers, therapists, coaches, and so forth, but also through the symbolic expressions of human relations that occur through myth, fairy tales, literature, art, music, film, television, advertising, the Internet, and many other forms of cultural transmission. We cannot choose our culture, nor do we enter and leave it at will. We are immersed in it from birth and define ourselves always within the context of the ground that it provides.

Michael White, the founding force, with David Epston, of *narrative therapy* (White, 2000, 2004; White & Epston, 1990), describes the identity of the person as emerging from

- Socially negotiated self narratives
- The impressions and imagination of others
- The performance of drama
- Dance, in play, in song, and in poetics
- Ritual, ceremony, and symbol
- Attire and in habits of life, and
- Personal and public documentation, dispersed through the inscriptions entered into community stories, into personal diaries, into correspondences in the form of letters and cards, into public

files in the form of profiles, assessments, and reports, and in the
longstanding tradition of autobiography. (White, 2004, p. 24)

According to White, these sources of identity lead to the possibility of
multiple identities (or multiple stories) that individuals may select in
order to make interpretive sense of and ascribe meaning to events in
their lives. He contrasts "intentional states" that emerge from these
social negotiations and lead to endorsements of particular beliefs, values,
or moral stances, with an individualistic psychological emphasis on "internal states" (e.g., drives, needs, biological deficits) that are often associated with attributions about health or illness. A goal of narrative therapy is to generate "externalizing conversations" with clients that move
them from perceiving their psychological difficulties as internally based
and personally pathological to an understanding of how their struggles
resonate with shared cultural themes and challenges. By breaking the
normative linkage of a problem to internal deficit (which is often what
White calls the *dominant story*), the narrative therapist frees the client to
explore alternative stories that are available within the cultural
"library." In this exploration, clients can locate a way of narrating their
experiences that feels more affirming and congruent with values that are
most uplifting and nurturing for them. At the same time, cultural narratives that operate at a less than obvious level, despite powerful influences
on behavior, can be made more explicit and recognizable.

White (2004) provides a creative and moving example of his intervention with an adolescent boy who had displayed violent outbursts toward his mother during arguments, including holding a knife to her
throat. Rather than focusing on the boy's "oppositional disorder" or his
"impulse control" deficit, White enlists first the father, then the grandfather, and eventually a male cousin, in a series of dialogues (with the boy
present) about relationships between men and women. Having established these other men's commitment to respect for women and their opposition to any form of aggression or physical intimidation, White continued to hold meetings in which these men talked about the negative
ways men can behave and the preferred alternatives men might employ
in their interactions with women. White dubbed these relatives of the
boy a "committee of men," who provided the boy with a collection of
more healthy narratives about male–female interactions. This committee
remained available to support and guide the boy toward more appropriate behavior. In addition to a decrease in the boy's negative behavior, the
father, grandfather, and cousin reported an improvement in their own relationships with the significant women in their lives.

The power of this intervention is that it does not perceive the person
simply as an isolated individual consisting of a set of internal working

parts that is susceptible to malfunction. Rather, narrative therapy understands this particular individual as a member of a male community linked across the generations to other males, all of whom share cultural understandings and practices of what it means to be male and of how males interact with women. We can treat the boy's difficulty with male aggression by accessing (or externalizing) more positive cultural narratives of male–female relations and helping the boy to integrate these narratives into his own personal identity. The role modeling, provided by his elders, is a powerful impetus for him to incorporate these more affirming visions into his rules of conduct. The positive effect that this intervention has on the other men is a perfect illustration of the embeddedness of all of the participants in each other's lives. They could not help the boy without experiencing the reverberations in their own lives. White (2004) writes:

> The appreciation of the cultural and historical character of the [alternate narratives available to us] has the effect of expanding therapeutic inquiry into the broad realms of living, providing people with new possibilities for drawing on and seeing through culture and history in their efforts to address their predicaments and their concerns. This gives people a basis for the development of some familiarity with ways of thinking and with practices of relationship that were previously little known, for options in self-formation previously unseen, and for the recognition of problem-solving skills not previously acknowledged or available. (p. 43)

All of the narrative advances I have just described—Pennebaker's emphasis on the meaning-making function of self-disclosure, King's work on the value of ambiguity and complexity in narrative accounts, Greenberg and Angus's demonstration of how emotional differentiation in narrative leads to better therapeutic outcomes, Luborsky and Crits-Christoph's careful delineation of relationship themes in narrative, and White's illustration of culturally constructed alternatives in narrative identity—map into the fundamental principles of the person-based psychology I have articulated (see the end of Chapter 6 for the enumeration of these principles). Each of these approaches shows a respect for the individual as an intentional and meaning-making entity. They recognize that the personality within the individual is a complex system that benefits from differentiation and flexibility rather than oversimplification and rigidity. They highlight the relational and cultural basis of the person and move us away from perspectives that see individuals as unanchored selves that move in and out of relationships and that are separable from the culture in which they are found. Finally, and critically, given that the linkage of personality psychology and psychotherapy is a theme of this book, these narrative investigations feature a variety of scientific methods, ranging from more laboratory-based and quantitative to naturalistic and interpretive approaches.

Edited volumes (e.g., Angus & McLeod, 2004) from which some of the above examples have been drawn, as well as the aforementioned American Psychological Association (APA) series on the narrative study of lives (Josselson et al., 2003; Lieblich, McAdams, & Josselson, 2004; McAdams, Josselson, & Lieblich, 2001) and a recent special issue of the *Journal of Personality* (Singer, 2004b) make a strong case for the sustained presence of this person-based psychology in a landscape dominated by cognitive science and biological perspectives.

Along with these significant pieces of work in the narrative area, I have sought in this volume to provide additional scientific justification for the value and application of a person-based psychology to psychotherapy. The struggle for how psychotherapy will be practiced is far from over and is likely to continue throughout this century. The particular approach I advocate in this volume, and the allied approaches to which it has referred, are truly engaged in a defense of therapy as a vehicle for exploration, understanding of self and other, and meaning making. On the other side of the battle lines are the forces of profit maximization, cost-containment, and efficiency that pressure therapy toward brief, symptom-based, technique-focused, pharmacologically oriented interventions. These latter influences are indeed moving us toward a depersonalized vision of therapy in which defective parts are identified, treated, or regulated. What is at stake is clearly more than schools and techniques of therapy, but how we propose to understand human nature and what aspects of the human being we will continue to value and respect. A person-based psychology sides with a view of human beings that embraces Shakespeare's words:

> What a piece of work is man! how noble in reason! how infinite
> in faculty! in form and moving how express and admirable!
> in action how like an angel! in apprehension how like a god! . . .
> (*Hamlet*, Act II, Scene ii, lines 315–319)

On this vision of human beings, the challenge to the therapist is clear—to proceed with due humility and resoluteness at the awesome task of engaging with and seeking to understand another person. Simultaneously, the challenge to individuals entering therapy is also clear and equally daunting—to risk vulnerability in the interest of uncovering the complexity and mystery of their own lives. In the interplay of therapist and client, we glimpse the dynamic tension of figure and ground that defines most fully the nature of the person. Depending on the vantage point we take at the moment, we can see either the defined figure of the individual person, asserting his or her free will to express a desire, declare a choice, or give voice to the deepest feelings of pain or joy, or we can shift our gaze and see the variegated context that engulfs both person and therapist in their reciprocal dialogue, the duties and obligations of work and family, or the political responsibilities of citizens.

In looking to Jennifer, the young woman on the verge of graduation from college, we witnessed her personal struggle with growing up and separating from her family, but we also saw how the societal response to her beauty threatened her capacity to accept and even gaze at her own image in a mirror.

In considering the successful businesswoman who struggled with her habit of shoplifting, we acknowledged the social costs of her action, not to mention the personal risk and guilt it engendered, and we also caught sight of the liberating function that her act of rebellion expressed in a despairing and abusive home.

In our encounters with Nell, we cited her moments of paralysis as signs of an underlying depression, but we also noted her struggles as belonging to a larger conflict that transcended her—a struggle between artistic expression and responsibility, about the need to stand at a mountain's edge or take the path that leads back home, or to see a white owl (that may not even really be there) burst free from the spiked fist of the tree that has concealed it.

Finally, in encountering Doug and Karen, we circled with them in their destructive dance, tracing their familiar steps to reveal one partner in her bedroom alone and the other outside in the night air, lit by the glow of a cigar, choked by hurt and fear too full to be given words.

For these individuals with whom I have worked in therapy, my goal has been to help them catch the fullest light of these images of self and other, and of the relationships that provide their context. In setting this goal, I have inevitably learned a great deal about each person and about myself, as well as about the *analytic third*, the synergic entity we mutually create. Person-based psychology and psychotherapy are centered in this willingness to remain open to the unfinished nature of human life, a process not of diagnosis but of discovery, not of classification but of curiosity, and ultimately, of reverence alongside revelation. In the spirit of Doug, the transactional man, and Karen, the woman of faith, a couple learning to meld their separate commitments to responsibility and relationship into a truly reciprocal marriage, a person-based psychology respects each person's capacity to take a stand in the world and to give ground for the stance of another, and finally to stand together, embedded in each other's life and in the larger world.

CONTACT INFORMATION FOR OBTAINING
INSTRUMENTS REFERRED TO IN THIS VOLUME

NEO PI-R—Psychological Assessment Resources
www.parinc.com

Personal Strivings Measure
Robert Emmons, PhD
Department of Psychology
University of California–Davis
Davis, CA 95616-8686
E-mail: raemmons@ucdavis.edu

Weinberger Adjustment Inventory—Short Form (WAI-SF)
Daniel Weinberger, PhD
Wellen Center
P.O. Box 22807
Beachwood, OH 44122
E-mail: Daw7@po.cwru.edu

Life Story and Identity Status Interviews (Appendices B and C)
Available in Josselson, R. (1996). *Revising herself: The story of women's identity from college to midlife* (pp. 262–272). New York: Oxford University Press.

Memory Coding Manual—McAdams—Life Story Interview
McAdams, D. P. (1988). *Power, intimacy, and the life story: Personological inquiries into identity.* New York: Guilford Press.

Dan P. McAdams, PhD
School of Education and Social Policy
Northwestern University
2120 Campus Drive
Evanston, IL 60208
E-mail: dmca@northwestern.edu

Foley Center for the Study of Lives
www.sesp.northwestern.edu/foley/

Singer and Blagov Scoring Manual
Jefferson A. Singer, PhD
Department of Psychology
Connecticut College
270 Mohegan Avenue
New London, CT 06320
E-mail: jasin@conncoll.edu

Thorne and McLean Scoring Manual
Avril Thorne, PhD
Psychology Department
University of California–Santa Cruz
Santa Cruz, CA 95064
E-mail: avril@ucsc.edu

THE HISTORICAL ROOTS
OF A PERSON-BASED PSYCHOLOGY

In this historical overview of the antecedents to contemporary person-based psychology, I present the story of Gordon Allport and his determined efforts to make personality psychology a science of the unique individual, with attention to both quantitative and phenomenological modes of inquiry. His commitment to this integrated approach demonstrates that the synthesis I have proposed in this volume may be traced to the very founding of personality psychology in the United States.

GORDON ALLPORT'S
"INVENTION OF PERSONALITY"

Gordon Allport (1897–1967) was one of the most prominent psychologists of the 20th century. He was a faculty member at Harvard University for nearly four decades, Chair of its Psychology Department, editor of personality and social psychology journals, president of the American Psychological Association (APA), and recipient of numerous honors and awards from various national and international scientific organizations. He is well-known for writing the first standard textbook of personality (Allport, 1937), pioneering the search for fundamental personality traits, developing a widely used personality test of values (Allport, Vernon, & Lindzey, 1970), and conducting groundbreaking work on the nature of prejudice (Allport, 1954), among many other contributions. His biographer, Ian Nicholson, notes that Allport's 1922 dissertation on personality traits was the first to be produced in the field of psychology, and his 1924 course on personality was certainly among the first to be taught in the United States. In a 1951 survey sponsored by the APA Division of Clinical and Abnormal Psychology, Allport ranked second only to Freud for the influence of his personality theories on clinical psychology (Nicholson, 2003). His influence, as mentor of generations of personality researchers and as spokesperson for the field of personality, spanned from the decade before the World War II to the Vietnam era.

Given these credentials, it would be helpful to explore the shaping influences on Allport's efforts to develop the academic field of personality (see Barenbaum, in press, for a recent and insightful analysis of the major psychological themes in Allport's life and their influence on his work). Allport was the

217

youngest of four sons of an Ohio physician. His mother was a highly religious woman who, along with her husband, strongly encouraged her sons to pursue their studies and become "men of character" who would take action for the betterment of others beyond themselves (Nicholson, 2003, p. 14). Allport's older brother Floyd went on to Harvard and developed his own successful career as a social psychologist. As Barenbaum (in press) documents, Allport recalled that his childhood years were filled with feelings of inferiority in relation to his dynamic and more confident older brothers. As the youngest brother, Gordon could not help feeling overshadowed by the various athletic, social, or academic successes of his brothers (Harold and Fayette in athletic and social realms, Floyd in scholarly pursuits). He was quite conscious of himself as more "tender-minded" than his brothers (more inclined toward aesthetic and religious concerns), and this sense of his difference was to play a substantial role in the crafting of his perspective on personality in the years ahead. Among the three older brothers, Allport could identify the most with Floyd, who was similarly inclined toward academic interests and distinctly more introverted than the other two.

Allport followed Floyd to Harvard and took up the study of social ethics (a kind of hybrid of social work, sociology, psychology, and moral philosophy). He involved himself in a number of service activities to impoverished youth outside the university, while also pursuing his religious life more ardently. After some poor grades initially, he intensified his studies and began to do extremely well. However, his early stumble left him with an enduring admiration for the rigor and high standards of Harvard.

According to Nicholson's analysis of these undergraduate years, Allport emerged with an appreciation for how the young fields of social work and psychology sought to apply scientific principles to human beings and the social conditions in which they lived. Besides social work's emphasis on "casework" and the individual client, Allport appreciated its shift in focus from the development of character steeped in an old-fashioned Victorian morality to the understanding and improvement of "personality." Still self-conscious about his association with more "feminized" studies and activities, Allport felt that the study of personality gave a more scientific and masculine quality to his interests:

> In the language of character, selfhood was achieved through surrender to a "higher" moral standard. In the new discourse of personality, selfhood was achieved through the realization of the self's own abilities. The true self of personality was not one of duty, honor, and self-sacrifice—terms that referred to a framework outside the self. Rather, personality was embedded in a language that reflected back on a more active and masculine self—"fascinating, stunning, attractive, magnetic, glowing, masterful, creative, dominant, forceful." (Nicholson, 2003, p. 37, quoting Susman, 1979, p. 217)

However, as Nicholson is careful to point out, the adoption of personality as a focus of social ethics and social work was not a rejection of moral commitment to social improvement but was instead a shift of emphasis. Sociology and psychology would change society by creating conditions that would allow individuals to flourish in expression of their true and best natures, as opposed to the previous generations' determination to suppress individual desires in favor of a greater social order. The mission was still to improve the lot of human beings, who too often were caught in lives of misery. However, now the goal was more liberating than restricting in its spirit. This transition from a character emphasis to a personality focus allowed Allport to integrate a sustained commitment to spiritual life with his increasing mastery of secular scientific ideas about human psychological processes.

> Humility and some mysticism, I felt, were indispensable for me: otherwise I would be victimized by my own arrogance. Arrogance in psychological theorizing has always antagonized me; I believe it is better to be tentative, eclectic, and humble. (Allport, 1968, p. 382)

Allport's choice to take up a missionary teaching post in Constantinople after his graduation only reinforces how important his religious and social calling was for him at that time. Still, after much soul searching during his year away, he gave up this post to return to Harvard on a fellowship and then began his doctoral work in psychology. Once again, his brother Floyd, now an instructor at Harvard, was influential in persuading him back toward his scientific pursuits. Floyd encouraged him to take up work on the systematic measurement of individual differences in personality. Following Floyd's suggestions, but recognizing his ambivalence about the limitations of experimental techniques, Allport produced in 1922 the first doctoral dissertation to examine personality traits with a variety of laboratory assessment methods.

Allport recounts a critical "self-defining memory" (see Chapter 4, this volume) from this period of his thesis work that is essential to understanding his approach to the study of personality. Allport traveled to Clark University to present his new personality research to a group of experimental psychologists, led by Edward Titchener, one of the towering figures of American psychology, who had trained at Oxford and earned his PhD under Wundt in Leipzig. After 2 days of presentations on sensory psychology, the graduate students had a brief opportunity to describe their research. Allport presented his work on personality and was met by dead silence and a scowl of disapproval from Titchener. Titchener later contacted his advisor at Harvard to ask why he had allowed Allport to work on the topic of personality. Allport called this horrifying experience "a turning point" (Allport, 1968, p. 386), and determined that he would never allow such narrow thinking to dissuade him from his larger project of developing a science of personality.

However, despite Allport's bravado and determination that he would not be affected by the narrow attitudes of the experimentalist hierarchy in American psychology, it seems apparent to students of his life and work that he could not abandon completely the traditions of measurement and scientific rigor that had formed his socialization into the academic world of psychology. Unlike Henry Murray, his future colleague in the Harvard psychology department and fellow champion of personality psychology, Allport always attempted to find his way within the mainstream of American psychology, endorsing for the most part its scientific standards and vocabulary. Murray, who had trained in the natural sciences and medicine, felt no indebtedness to academic psychology and often openly criticized its imitative efforts to appear more "scientific." He once wrote that academic psychology

> not only failed to bring light to the great, hauntingly recurrent problems, but it
> has no intention, one is shocked to realize, of attempting to investigate them.
> (Murray, 1935/1981, p. 339, cited in Anderson, 1990, p. 319)

Allport was of a different and more conciliatory temperament. He was increasingly frustrated with the experimental and behaviorist domination of psychology, but he continued to seek ways to work within its power structure. Perhaps, as Barenbaum (in press) suggests, he could never fully break from the experimental emphasis that his brother Floyd had so strongly modeled for him.

One more pivotal formative influence requires mention before I turn to Allport's seminal textbook. After receiving his degree, Allport spent the next 2 years, 1922–1924, in Germany on a Sheldon Traveling Fellowship. He called this experience his "second intellectual dawn" (Allport, 1968, p. 386) to accompany the awakening he received when he came to Harvard. Critical to our person-based interest is Allport's exposure to the personalistic psychology of William Stern and the psychology of types of Eduard Spranger, as well as the gestalt psychology of Wertheimer and Kohler. The work of Stern and Spranger espoused a *verstehen* perspective mentioned in Chapter 1—an emphasis on a nonreductive understanding of human experience. This perspective traced its origin to a Kantian and Romantic sensibility that rejected an associational or atomistic vision of psychology in favor of a concern with studying individuals in contexts that reveal intention and meaning. Anticipating by several decades the cognitive revolution in American psychology, this wave of German psychology shared a concern with a priori categories of knowledge and perception. *Gestalt* psychologists, working out of a more empirical perspective, were able to verify a number of these more philosophical ideas through a series of simple but elegant experiments. These ideas and research influenced all branches of psychology, including the cognitive-developmental theories of Piaget, the "behavior is a function of the person and the environment" framework of Kurt Lewin and his followers in social psychology, and the early memory schema work of Frederick Bartlett at Cambridge University.

For Allport, German psychology's concern with the integrity of the individual's unique experience of a phenomenon had a profound effect on his developing ideas about personality. From this work Allport developed his famous *idiographic versus nomothetic* distinction in studying the person, borrowing these phrases from the German philosopher, Windelband (1894/1998, cited in Lamiell, 2003). In a probing historical and philosophical account of the usage of these two terms, Lamiell (2003) traces the original meaning of these terms to a speech by Windelband on the occasion of his installation as the rector of the University of Strassburg in 1894. Since these two terms are often used loosely in personality courses and discussions, it is worth quoting Lamiell's translation of Windelband's introduction of them:

> So we may say that the empirical sciences seek in knowledge of reality either the general in the form of the natural law or the particular in the historically determined form [*Gestalt*]. They consider in one part the ever-enduring form, in the other part the unique content, determined within itself, of an actual happening. The one comprise sciences of law, the other sciences of events; the former teach us what always is [*was immer ist*], the latter what once was [*was einmal war*]. If one may resort to neologisms, it can be said that *scientific thought is in the one case nomothetic, in the other idiographic.* (Windelband, 1894/1998, p. 13, cited in Lamiell, 2003, p. 180; emphasis added by Lamiell)

If we think then about the idiographic perspective as the study of "what once was," it is fundamentally an investigation into the unique confluence of specific events and forces that have produced a nonrepeatable historical event. Nomothetic study would be the identification of general laws that transcend historical happenings to provide immutable explanations that would not vary from one occurrence to the next. (As Lamiell carefully points out, this original usage of *nomothetic* has been transformed in contemporary psychology into a looser and technically inaccurate rendering that simply means "accounts of personality that rely on aggregation rather than the study of the unique individual").

In his pursuit of a new personality psychology, Allport was highly swayed by strains of German thought and psychology that emphasized the idiographic concern for unique phenomenological experience. According to Allport's way of defining *idiographic* in terms of personality research, idiographic approaches do not attempt to explain the individual by locating a particular response of the individual on a continuum of responses generated by similar individuals. To do so glosses over the unique meaning and circumstances associated with this response for that particular individual. Idiographic approaches seek to study a given response only in the context of that individual's particular repertoire of responses in similar situations and to similar stimuli. "Differential psychology" approaches are not concerned with the individual in this way, but more with locating individuals in relation to each other in the service of a larger construct, such as intelligence, friendliness, or aggression. Allport wrote:

> Mental tests are a typical achievement of differential psychology. Individuals are discovered to vary "normally" in some function (such as intelligence, perseveration, or introversion), and the degree of a person's variation above or

below the mean is considered to be his score. It is quite clear that the chief interest is one elementary attribute at a time. The peculiar patterning of attributes within the single person is not considered. (1937, p. 9)

Importantly, one of the great innovations in recent personality assessment, whether in the application of the Minnesota Multiphasic Personality Inventory (MMPI) or the Revised NEO Personality Inventory (NEO PI-R), has been an increased emphasis on the *patterns* of measured attributes that distinguish subgroups of individuals from each other. Though not the individualized patterns that Allport urged researchers to identify, this work is far less atomistic than the original reliance on a single construct, such as dominance or self-consciousness, to divide up individuals.

We should note that in embracing a scientific psychology oriented toward the person, Allport also saw the limitations of a psychoanalytic perspective, which on the surface might have seemed more embracing of individuality than experimental psychology. He argued that psychoanalysis, in its reduction of all psychological motivation to two fundamental motives of sex and aggression, was in its own way just as limiting as an emphasis on behaviorist or learning principles. Similar to his critique of mechanistic psychology for its "empty organism" view of human beings (Allport, 1955, p. 100), Allport saw the deterministic position of psychoanalysis as a rejection of the "functional autonomy" of much of human motivation. He felt that the particular configuration of the individual's traits in combination with specific situational factors yielded a unique set of perceptions and accompanying actions that, while ultimately lawful, were not a simple function of one or two dominant motives. In this sense, Allport was much more favorable to the influence of conscious forces, such as wishes, strivings, and values, on an individual's behavior. The current work of Mischel and Shoda (Mischel, Shoda, & Mendoza-Denton, 2002) on their cognitive–affective personality system (CAPS) argues for exactly this kind of situation-contingent dynamic process as the individual responds to a given stimulus in a particular setting, and it is no coincidence that an important summary of their theory begins with an allusion to Allport's work (Mishcel & Shoda, 1999; see also Zuroff, 1986, for the linkage between Allport's and Mischel's view on trait-context contingencies).

Allport's textbook (Allport, 1937), embracing both general principles of psychology and idiographic pursuit of the unique individual, set the standard for personality textbooks for the next 25 years, but there is one more critical contribution made by Allport in this period that I would like to highlight. I have mentioned his colleague Henry Murray, who directed the Psychological Clinic at Harvard University during Allport's time on the faculty. Murray should be familiar to most students of psychology for his development of the concept of diverse psychogenic needs, such as the need for achievement, need for dominance, and the need for affiliation, as well as the Thematic Apperception Test (TAT), which he created with Christiana Morgan, as a projective test to record these needs (Murray, 1943). In 1938, Murray, assisted by the many collaborators from his clinic, published his magnum opus, *Explorations in Personality*. This work was breathtaking in its efforts to take up the concern for individuality that was at the heart of Allport's new person-based personality psychology. Using his own term, *personology* (see Chapter 1, this volume) to distinguish his interest in the person from the individual-differences perspective of most personality psychologists, Murray studied small numbers of participants intensively, collecting well over 30 hours of data per individual. These data combined experimental tests, self-report inventories, projective tests, behavioral observation, autobiographical writings, and many other techniques, all recorded by a team of researchers. Once the data were compiled, a smaller "Diagnostic Council" of more senior researchers, led by Murray himself, attempted to develop a formulation of the individual that would be integrative and comprehensive in its account of the individual's history, motivation, and likely future challenges and conflicts. Though in no way doctrinaire, these formulations drew widely on psychodynamic concepts borrowed from Freud and Jung, as well as Murray's own nascent personality theory.

Murray's impact on personality psychology has been extensive, as has been the impact of many of the original authors of *Explorations in Personality*, including Erik Erikson (who, in the brief time he was with Murray, was still known as Erik Homburger), Robert White, Donald MacKinnon, Saul Rosenzweig, and Nevitt Sanford. To this list should be added other colleagues and students over his years at Harvard—Silvan Tomkins, Brewster Smith, David McClelland, and David Winter, among others. Any check through an index of a typical personality textbook will indicate that these researchers' contributions underscore the rich and substantial legacy of Murray's influence. Murray's work directly lives on in McAdams's life-story theory of identity, which forms the heart of Chapter 4, this volume, as well as in the psychobiographical work of researchers such as Elms (1994), Runyan (1982, 1997), and Schultz (2002). This research is characterized by not only a critical focus on the individual but also an interest in fantasy, dream, memory, symbolism, and myth, all aspects of personality that seldom receive attention from the individual-differences perspective. In honor of Murray's contribution to personality psychology, Division 8 of the American Psychological Association (the Division of Personality and Social Psychology) presents an annual Henry A. Murray Award to the personality psychologist who has best exemplified the ongoing tradition of personological research.

Besides working alongside Allport for over three decades, Murray is critical to the story of the origin of person-based psychology because of an incident that exemplified Allport's endorsement of the middle way in personality psychology. As Anderson (1990), Nicholson (2003), and Robinson (1992) all recount, Murray came up for reappointment at Harvard in 1936. The members of the committee to evaluate his status included Edwin Boring, the experimentalist and historian of psychology, Karl Lashley, one of the first great physiological psychologists, three other faculty members from the administration and other departments, the President of Harvard University, James Bryant Conant, and Gordon Allport. Not surprisingly, Boring and Lashley accused Murray of inferior research standards and loose, undisciplined ideas. Allport, despite his own personal reservations over the psychodynamic emphases of Murray work, stood up for the new approach to personality represented by Murray's efforts. When the vote ended up deadlocked, Allport applied some pressure by bringing up a recent invitation he had received to move to another institution (on the other side, Lashley made a more overt threat to leave if Murray were retained). Pleading Murray's case,

Allport wrote:

> I earnestly hope that you will not now permit the humanistic tradition in psychology at Harvard to be imperiled and destroyed. The critical standards of the "exact sciences," admirable in their own right, are not catholic enough in outlook to serve as the norm for the newer science of the human mind. (1936, cited in Anderson, 1990, p. 325)

Ultimately, Conant broke the tie and did indeed reappoint Murray, though not with tenure, and only to an associate professor rank. However, Allport's intervention had saved Murray's status at Harvard and allowed the work that led to *Explorations in Personality* to continue. Allport acted on principle, but also strategically; having Murray in his department for years to come always made his own humanistic leanings seem just a bit more moderate next to the more sweeping and discursive approach that characterized Murray's contributions.

Runyan (1997) sums up this founding period in the history of person-based personality psychology:

> When personality psychology crystallized as a field in the 1930s with the seminal books by Allport (1937) and Murray (1938), it could be seen as reacting against the sterile formalisms of academic psychophysics, and as an effort to integrate the rigor of academic methods with the understanding of persons and lives. In the turn away from the study of lives in the 1950s and 1960s, there was a far greater emphasis on the "hard" tradition measurement and experimentation, with a decline of interest in the "softer" issues of studying whole persons and in developing general theories of personality. (1997, p. 63)

SINCE ALLPORT

This image of Allport as the provident Arthur, and Murray as the reckless Lancelot, in the Camelot days of Harvard personality psychology is the place where I would like to leave this "origin myth" of a person-based psychology. The intervening history until the last decade, as hinted at by Runyan, was of a difficult and often losing battle against the forces of behaviorism and psychoanalysis. McAdams (1997) beautifully documents these subsequent decades in which personality psychology lost sight of the person in favor of constructs such as the "authoritarian personality" (Adorno, Frenkel-Brunswik, Levinson, & Sanford, 1950), field independence (Witkin, 1950), or locus of control (Rotter, 1966). These construct approaches were a partial response to the failure of personality psychology to converge around a "grand theory" and its subsequent confusion, caused by a proliferation of nonfalsifiable pronouncements about the fundamental motives and dynamics of human beings. Unfortunately, construct psychology's escape from grand theories also meant a lack of concern with an integrative person-based psychology that had been at the heart of Allport's project.

Another significant development in personality psychology at midcentury and well into the 1970s was the "Third Wave" or humanistic psychology critique of the dominant paradigms of behaviorism and psychoanalysis. In an insightful history of humanistic psychology, Moss (2001, p. 14) identifies the years 1954–1973 as the "golden years of the humanistic psychology movement." The former date marked the year that Maslow created a mailing list for persons interested in the study of topics related to personal growth and self-actualization, while the latter date heralded the publication of the first academic textbook detailing humanistic psychology and research (Misiak & Sexton, 1973). In addition to Maslow (1954/1987), Rogers (1951), Fromm (1941), and Frankl (1963), among many other humanistic scholars and researchers, sought ways to retrieve a sense of meaning and integrative wholeness from the reductive perspectives of behaviorism and psychoanalysis. Their interest in the self's continual development and potential for growth over the life span was very much in line with Allport's own humanist vision. However, in their determination to distance their theories and research from the positivist experimental tradition, humanistic psychologists often found themselves at the periphery of American academic psychology. Although highly influential on the practice of therapy and in the thinking of the general public about issues of personal growth and self-actualization, their qualitative and phenomenological methods (see Wertz, 2001) often failed to interest and persuade quantitatively oriented personality psychologists (the great exception here was Rogers, who was much more inclined toward empirical research). Some writers have also documented the excesses and self-indulgent directions that some followers of humanistic doctrines ended up pursuing (Milton, 2001). In some ways, the splitting of humanistic psychology from the mainstream of personality psychology was Allport's greatest fear. The very basis of his approach had been a synthesis of a concern for the whole person with advances in experimental psychology.

If the construct personality psychology of the 1950s and 1960s came under attack from the grander theories of humanistic psychology, it received a devastating critique from the experimental direction when Walter Mischel (1968) reviewed the general inability of personality inventories to predict behavior at anything better than a 9–10% rate. Despite spirited defenses by Bem and Allen (1974), Block (1977), and Epstein (1979), personality psychology as a field, let alone person-based personality psychology, seemed to be in a continued decline. Fewer and fewer doctoral programs in psychology offered a personality track, and social psychologists dominated the major journal in the field, the *Journal of Personality and Social Psychology*. As personality psychology faded in influence, cognitive psychology was powerfully ascendant. Its influence quickly pervaded social psychology, creating the field of social cognition, which has been the leading area of research for social psychologists since the early 1980s.

Ironically, social cognition, with its emphasis on interpretive structures such as schemas, prototypes, and scripts, found its way back to enduring cognitive–affective patterns within the individual, sometimes referred to as person or self-schemas (Markus, 1977). Researchers such as Abelson (Schank & Abelson, 1977), Kihlstrom (1981), and J. L. Singer (Singer & Kolligian, 1987), all influenced by the writings of Silvan Tomkins (1962, 1963, 1979, 1987), who made integrative links between cognition and affect (see a discussion of his work in Chapter 4, this volume), encouraged social cognition researchers to incorporate personality, affective, and motivational influences into their models. At the same time in the early 1980s, with the advent of the Big Five and its associated instruments (see Chapter 2, this volume), individual-differences psychology experienced a leap in sophistication and was finally able to shake off the negative collar applied to it by Mischel's earlier work. The next piece of this puzzle was the surge of interest in narrative as a unifying object of study across the social sciences and humanities. As I documented in Chapter 4, this volume, narrative allows for the integration of all aspects of the person in the context of sociocultural factors that in large part shape the identity of individuals. Finally, from outside the mainstream of academic psychology but increasingly forging theoretic, empirical, and clinical linkages, was the work of relational and social-constructive psychoanalysis, as typified by Mitchell (2000) and Ogden (1994), the focus of Chapter 5, this volume.

In drawing on each of these perspectives—trait/individual differences, social-cognitive processes (that include affect and motivation), narrative identity, and the relational/contextual understanding of the individual—we have found our way back to Allport's vision of a person-based psychology. As evidenced by a recent special issue of the *Journal of Personality* on narrative identity (Singer, 2004b) and the ongoing edited volumes on narrative published by the American Psychological Association (Josselson et al., 2003; Lieblich, McAdams, & Josselson, 2004; McAdams et al., 2001), an expanding group of researchers have re-embraced the study of the individual as a critical component of personality psychology.

In allegiance with the original vision of personality psychology that Allport proclaimed with his 1937 textbook, this group of researchers advocates a middle way that accepts the best aspects of experimental psychology but combines this nomothetic approach with idiographic and integrative methods. In doing so, its methods reflect an underlying attitude about the nature of the person, which is open, ecumenical, and committed to a respect for the power of both the individual will and the sociocultural milieu. While honoring the person, it pointedly avoids the antiscience rhetoric of the more extreme aspects of the Third Wave humanistic psychology movement described earlier. With this resurgence of a person-based personality psychology, it is an opportune time to make the bridge between this research approach and practitioners of therapy who seek to understand the whole person, and who valorize meaning, integration, and moral purpose in their therapeutic work.

References

Adler, A. (1927). *Understanding human nature.* New York: Greenberg.

Adler, A. (1930). *The neurotic constitution.* New York: Dodd, Mead.

Adorno, T. W., Frenkel-Brunswik, E., Levinson, D. J., & Sanford, R. N. (1950). *The authoritarian personality.* New York: Harper & Brothers.

Ainsworth, M. D. S. (1989). Attachments beyond infancy. *American Psychologist, 44,* 709–716.

Ainsworth, M. D. S., Blehar, M. C., Waters, E., & Wall, S. (1978). *Patterns of attachment: A psychological study of the strange situation.* Hillsdale, NJ: Erlbaum.

Aldwin, C. M., & Levensen, M. R. (1994). Aging and personality assessment. In M. P. Lawton & J. A. Teresi (Eds.), *Annual review of gerontology and geriatrics* (Vol. 14, pp. 182–209). New York: Springer.

Alexander, I. (1990). *Personology: Method and content in personality and psychobiography.* Durham, NC: Duke University Press.

Allport, G. W. (1937). *Personality: A psychological interpretation.* New York: Holt, Rinehart & Winston.

Allport, G. W. (1954). *The nature of prejudice.* Cambridge, MA: Addison-Wesley.

Allport, G. W. (1955). *Becoming: Basic considerations for a psychology of personality.* New Haven, CT: Yale University Press.

Allport, G. W. (1968). *The person in psychology: Selected essays by Gordon W. Allport.* Boston: Beacon Press.

Allport, G. W., & Odbert, H. S. (1936). Trait-names, a psychological study. *Psychological Monographs, 47*(1, Whole No. 211).

Allport, G. W., Vernon, P., & Lindzey, G. (1970). *Manual for the study of values* (3rd ed.). Boston: Houghton Mifflin.

Anderson, J. W. (1990). The life of Henry Murray: 1893–1988. In A. I. Rabin, R. A. Zucker, R. A. Emmons, & S. Frank (Eds.), *Studying persons and lives* (pp. 304–334). New York: Springer.

Angus, L. E., & McLeod, J. (Eds.). (2004). *The handbook of narrative and psychotherapy: Practice, theory, and research.* Thousand Oaks, CA: Sage.

Ansbacher, H. L. (1947). Adler's place today in the psychology of memory. *Journal of Personality, 3,* 197–207.

Ansbacher, H. L. (1973). Adler's interpretation of early recollections: Historical account. *Journal of Individual Psychology, 29,* 135–145.

Asendorpf, J. B., & van Aken, M. A. (1999). Resilient, overcontrolled, and undercontrolled personality prototypes in childhood: Replicability, predictive power, and the trait–type issue. *Journal of Personality and Social Psychology, 77,* 815–832.

Atkinson, J. W., Heyns, R. W., & Veroff, J. (1954). The effect of experimental arousal of the affiliation motive on thematic apperception. *Journal of Abnormal and Social Psychology, 49,* 405–410.

Baars, B. (2002). The conscious access hypothesis. *Trends in Cognitive Sciences, 6,* 47–52.

Bakan, D. (1966). *The duality of human existence: Isolation and communion in western man.* Boston: Beacon Press.

Baldonado, A. (Producer). (2004, March 17). *Fresh Air* [Radio broadcast]. New York: National Public Radio.

Banaji, M. R. (2001). Implicit attitudes can be measured. In H. L. Roediger & J. S. Nairne (Eds.), *The nature of remembering: Essays in honor of Robert G. Crowder* (pp. 117–150). Washington DC: American Psychological Association.

Bandura, A. (1999). Social cognitive theory of personality. In L. A. Pervin & O. P. John (Eds.), *Handbook of personality: Theory and research* (2nd ed., pp. 154–196). New York: Guilford Press.

Bandura, A. (2001). The changing face of psychology at the dawning of a globalization era. *Canadian Psychology, 42,* 12–24.

Bandura, A., Barbarnelli, C., Caprara, G. V., & Pastorelli, C. (1996). Mechanisms of moral disengagement in the exercise of moral agency. *Journal of Personality and Social Psychology, 71,* 364–374.

Barenbaum, N. B. (in press). Four, two, or one?: Gordon Allport and the unique personality. In W. T. Schultz (Ed.), *Handbook of psychobiography.* New York: Oxford University Press.

Bargh, J. A. (1997). The automaticity of everyday life. In R. S. Wyer, Jr. (Ed.), *Advances in social cognition* (Vol. 10, pp. 1–61). Mahwah, NJ: Erlbaum.

Barrett, L. F. (1997). The relationships among momentary emotion experiences, personality descriptions, and retrospective ratings of emotion. *Personality and Social Psychology Bulletin, 23,* 1100–1110.

Barrick, M. R., & Mount, M. K. (1991). The Big Five personality dimensions and job performance: A meta-analysis. *Personnel Psychology, 44,* 1–26.

Bartholomew, K., & Horowitz, L. M. (1991). Attachment styles among young adults: A test of a model. *Journal of Personality and Social Psychology, 61,* 226–244.

Bauer, J. J., & Bonanno, G. A. (2001). Continuity and discontinuity: Bridging one's past and present in stories of conjugal bereavement. *Narrative Inquiry, 11,* 123–158.

Baumeister, R. (1986). *Identity: Cultural change and the struggle for the self.* New York: Oxford University Press.

Baumeister, R. (1987). How the self became a problem: A psychological review of historical research. *Journal of Personality and Social Psychology, 52,* 163–176.

Behrends, R. S., & Blatt, S. J. (2003). Psychodynamic assessment. In J. S. Wiggins (Ed.), *Paradigms of personality assessment* (pp. 226–245). New York: Guilford Press.

Bellah, R. N., Sullivan, W. M., Swidler, A., & Tipton, S. M. (1985). *Habits of the heart: Individualism and commitment in American life.* Berkeley: University of California Press.

Bem, D. J., & Allen, A. (1974). On predicting some of the people some of the time: The search for cross-situational consistencies in behavior. *Psychological Review, 81,* 506–520.

Benjamin, J. (1998). *Shadow of the other: Intersubjectivity and gender in psychoanalysis.* New York: Routledge.

Benjamin, J. (1999). An outline of intersubjectivity: The development of recognition. *Psychoanalytic Psychology, 7*(Suppl.), 33–46. (Original work published 1990)

Beutler, L. E., & Groth-Marnat, G. (2003). *Integrative assessment of adult personality* (2nd ed.). New York: Guilford Press.

Blagov, P. S., & Singer, J. A. (2004). Four dimensions of self-defining memories (specificity, meaning, content, and affect) and their relationships to self-restraint, distress, and repressive defensiveness. *Journal of Personality, 72,* 481–511.

Blaney, P. H. (1986). Affect and memory: A review. *Psychological Bulletin, 99,* 229–246.

Blatt, S. J. (1990). Interpersonal relatedness and self-definition: Two personality configurations and their implications for psychopathology and psychotherapy. In J. L. Singer (Ed.), *Repression and dissociation* (pp. 299–335). Chicago: University of Chicago Press.

Block, J. (1977). Advancing the psychology of personality: Paradigmatic shift or improving the quality of research. In D. Magnusson & N. S. Endler (Eds.), *Personality at the crossroads: Current issues in interactional psychology* (pp. 37–64). Hillsdale, NJ: Erlbaum.

Bluck, S., & Gluck, J. (2004). Making things better and learning a lesson: "Wisdom of experience" narratives across the lifespan. *Journal of Personality, 72,* 543–572.

Bluck, S., & Habermas, T. (2000). The life story schema. *Motivation and Emotion, 24,* 121–147.

Book, H. (2004). The CCRT approach to working with patient narratives in psychodynamic psychotherapy. In L. E. Angus & J. McLeod (Eds.), *Handbook of narrative and psychotherapy: Practice, theory, and research* (pp. 71–86). Thousand Oaks, CA: Sage.

Bornat, J. (2002). Reminiscence and oral history: Comparisons across parallel universes. In J. D. Webster & B. K. Haight (Eds.), *Critical advances in reminiscence work: From theory to application* (pp. 33–43). New York: Springer Co.

Bouchard, T. J., Jr., Lykken, D. T., McGue, M., Segal, N. L., & Tellegen, A. (1990). Sources of human psychological differences: The Minnesota study of twins reared apart. *Science, 250,* 223–228.

Bowlby, J. (1944). Forty-four juvenile thieves: Their characters and home life. *International Journal of Psychoanalysis, 25,* 19–52, 107–127.

Bowlby, J. (1951). *Maternal care and mental health* (WHO Monograph No. 2). Geneva: World Health Organization.

Bowlby, J. (1969). *Attachment and loss: Vol. 1. Attachment.* New York: Basic Books.

Bowlby, J. (1973). *Attachment and loss: Vol. 2. Separation: Anxiety and anger.* New York: Basic Books.

Bowlby, J. (1980). *Attachment and loss: Vol. 3. Loss.* New York: Basic Books.

Boyatzis, R. E. (1973). Affiliation motivation. In D. C. McClelland & R. S. Steele (Eds.), *Human motivation: A book of readings* (pp. 252–276). Morristown, NJ: General Learning Press.

Briggs, J. L. (1970). *Never in anger: Portrait of an Eskimo family.* Cambridge, MA: Harvard University Press.

Briggs, J. L. (1998). *Inuit morality play.* New Haven, CT: Yale University Press.

Brown, J. D. (1998). *The self.* New York: McGraw-Hill.

Bruhn, A. R. (1984). The use of early memories as a projective technique. In P. McReynolds & C. J. Chelume (Eds.), *Advances in psychological assessment* (Vol. 6, pp. 109–150). San Francisco: Jossey-Bass.

Bruhn, A. R. (1990). *Earliest childhood memories: Vol. 1. Theory and application to clinical practice.* New York: Praeger.

Bruner, J. (1990). *Acts of meaning.* Cambridge, MA: Harvard University Press.

Buss, D. M. (1995). Evolutionary psychology: A new paradigm for psychological science. *Psychological Inquiry, 6,* 1–30.

Buss, D. M. (1996). Social adaptation and the five major factors of personality. In J. S. Wiggins (Ed.), *The five-factor model of personality: Theoretical perspectives* (pp. 180–207). New York: Guilford Press.

Butcher, J. N. (2002). *Clinical personality assessment: Practical approaches* (2nd Ed.). New York: Oxford University Press.

Butler, R. N. (1980). The life review: An unrecognized bonanza. *International Journal of Aging and Human Development, 12,* 35–38.

Cantor, N., & Langston, C. A. (1989). Ups and downs of life tasks in a life transition. In L. A. Pervin (Ed.), *Goal concepts in personality and social psychology* (pp. 127–167). Hillsdale, NJ: Erlbaum.

Cantor, N., Norem, J. K., Niedenthal, P. M., Langston, C. A., & Brower, A. M. (1987). Life tasks, self-concept ideals, and cognitive strategies in a life transition. *Journal of Personality and Social Psychology, 53,* 1178–1191.

Carver, C. S., & Scheier, M. F. (1981). *Attention and self-regulation: A control theory approach to human behavior.* New York: Springer-Verlag.

Carver, C. S., & Scheier, M. F. (1998). *On the self-regulation of behavior.* New York: Cambridge University Press.

Carver, C. S., & Scheier, M. F. (1999). Stress, coping, and self-regulating processes. In L. A. Pervin & O. P. John (Eds.), *Handbook of personality: Theory and research* (2nd ed., pp. 553–575). New York: Guilford Press.

Carver, C. S., & Scheier, M. F. (2004). *Perspectives on personality* (5th ed.). Boston: Allyn & Bacon.

Cash, T. F. (2002). Women's body images. In G. M. Wingood & R. J. DiClemente (Eds.), *Handbook of women's sexual and reproductive health: Issues in women health* (pp. 175–194). New York: Kluwer Academic/Plenum Publishers.

Caspi, A., & Roberts, B. W. (1999). Personality continuity and change across the life course. In L. A. Pervin & O. P. John (Eds.), *Handbook of personality: Theory and practice* (2nd ed., pp. 300–326). New York: Guilford Press.

Cattell, R. B. (1946). *The description and measurement of personality*. Yonkers, NY: World Book.

Cattell, R. B., Eber, H. W., & Tatsuoka, M. M. (1970). *The handbook for the Sixteen Personality Factor Questionnaire*. Champaign, IL: Institute for Personality and Ability Testing.

Chodorow, N. (1999). *The power of feelings: Personal meaning in psychoanalysis, gender, and culture*. New Haven, CT: Yale University Press.

Churchill, S. D., & Wertz, F. J. (2001). An introduction to phenomenological research in psychology: Historical, conceptual, and methodological foundations. In K. J. Schneider, J. F. T. Bugental, & J. F. Pierson (Eds.), *The handbook of humanistic psychology: Leading edges in theory, research, and practice* (pp. 247–262). Thousand Oaks, CA: Sage.

Clark, L. A., & Livesley, W. J. (1994). Two approaches to identifying dimensions of personality disorder: Convergence on the five-factor model. In P. T. Costa, Jr. & T. A. Widiger (Eds.), *Personality disorders and the five-factor model of personality* (pp. 261–278). Washington, DC: American Psychological Association.

Conway, M. A., & Pleydell-Pearce, C. W. (2000). The construction of autobiographical memories in the self-memory system. *Psychological Review, 107*, 261–288.

Conway, M. A., Singer, J. A., & Tagini, A. (2004). The self and autobiographical memory: Correspondence and coherence. *Social Cognition, 22*, 491–529.

Costa, P. T., Jr., & McCrae, R. R. (1988). From catalog to classification: Murray's needs and the five-factor nodel. *Journal of Personality and Social Psychology, 55*, 258–265.

Costa, P. T., Jr., & McCrae, R. R. (1990). Personality disorders and the five-factor model of personality. *Journal of Personality Disorders, 4*, 362–371.

Costa, P. T., Jr., & McCrae, R. R. (1992). *NEO-PI-R and NEO-FFI: Professional manual*. Odessa, FL: Psychological Assessment Resources.

Costa, P. T., Jr., & McCrae, R. R. (1998). *Manual supplement for the NEO PI-R*. Odessa, FL: Psychological Assessment Resources.

Costa, P. T., Jr., & Piedmont, R. L. (2003). Multivariate assessment: NEO PI-R profiles of Madeleine G. In J. S. Wiggins (Ed.), *Paradigms of personality assessment* (pp. 262–280). New York: Guilford Press.

Costa, P. T., Jr., & Widiger, T. A. (Eds.). (2002). *Personality disorders and the five-factor model of personality* (2nd ed.). Washington DC: American Psychological Association.

Crits-Christoph, P., Demorest, A., Muenz, L., & Baranckie, K. (1994). Consistency of interpersonal themes for patients in psychotherapy. *Journal of Personality, 62,* 499–526.

Crits-Christoph, P., & Lubortsky, L. (1998). Changes in CCRT pervasiveness during psychotherapy. In L. Lubortsky & P. Crits-Christoph (Eds.), *Understanding transference: The core conflictual relationship theme method* (pp. 151–164). Washington, DC: American Psychological Association.

Cushman, P. (1995). *Constructing the self, constructing America: A cultural history of psychotherapy.* Reading, MA: Addison-Wesley.

Davis, P. J., & Schwartz, G. E. (1987). Repression and the inaccessibility of affective memories. *Journal of Personality and Social Psychology, 52,* 155–162.

Debats, D. L., Drost, J., & Hansen, P.. (1995). Experiences of meaning in life: A combined qualitative and quantitative approach. *British Journal of Psychology, 86,* 359–375.

Demorest, A. (1995). The personal script as a unit of analysis for the study of personality. *Journal of Personality, 63,* 569–591.

Demorest, A.P., & Alexander, I.E. (1992). Affective scripts as organizers of personal experience. *Journal of Personality, 60,* 645–663.

Dickens, C. (1962). *David Copperfield.* New York: Signet Classics. (Original works published 1869)

Digman, J. M. (1989). Five robust trait dimensions: Development, stability, and utility [Special issue: Longterm stability and change in personality]. *Journal of Personality, 57,* 195–214.

Dilthey, W. (1976). The development of hermeneutics. In H. P. Rickman (Ed.), *W. Dilthey: Selected writings.* Cambridge, UK: Cambridge University Press. (Original work published 1900)

Dilthey, W. (1977). *Descriptive psychology and human understanding.* The Hague, The Netherlands: Martinus Nijhoff. (Original work published 1894)

Dreyfus, H. (1991). *Being-in-the-world: A commentary on Heidegger's* Being and Time. Cambridge, MA: MIT Press.

Elkind, D. (1981). *Children and adolescents* (3rd ed.). New York: Oxford University Press.

Elliot, A. J., Sheldon, K. M., & Church, M. A. (1997). Avoidance personal goals and subjective well-being. *Personality and Social Psychology Bulletin, 23,* 915–927.

Elms, A. (1994). *Uncovering lives: The uneasy alliance of biography and psychology.* New York: Oxford University Press.

Emmons, R. A. (1986). Personal strivings: An approach to personality and subjective well-being. *Journal of Personality and Social Psychology, 51,* 1058–1068.

Emmons, R. A. (1989). The personal striving approach to personality. In L. A. Pervin (Ed.), *Goal concepts in personality and social psychology* (pp. 87–126). Hillsdale, NJ: Erlbaum.

Emmons, R. A. (1997). Motives and life goals. In R. Hogan, J. Johnson, & S. Briggs (Eds.), *Handbook of personality psychology* (pp. 485–512). San Diego: Academic Press.

Emmons, R. A. (1999). *The psychology of ultimate concerns: Motivation and spirituality in personality.* New York: Guilford Press.

Emmons, R. A., & King, L. A. (1988). Conflict among personal strivings: Immediate and long-term implications for psychological and physical well-being. *Journal of Personality and Social Psychology, 54,* 1040–1048.

Emmons, R. A., & McAdams, D. P. (1991). Personal strivings and motive dispositions: Exploring the links. *Personality and Social Psychology Bulletin, 17,* 648–654.

Entwisle, D. R. (1972). To dispel fantasies about fantasy-based measures of achievement motivation. *Psychological Bulletin, 77,* 377–391.

Epstein, S. (1979). The stability of behavior: 1. On predicting most of the people much of the time. *Journal of Personality and Social Psychology, 37,* 1097–1126.

Epstein, S. (1984). The stability of behavior across time and situations. In R. A. Zucker, J. Aronoff, & A. I. Rabin (Eds.), *Personality and the prediction of behavior* (pp. 209–268). New York: Academic Press.

Erikson, E.H. (1959). *Identity and the life cycle: Selected papers.* Oxford, UK: International Universities Press.

Erikson, E. H. (1963). *Childhood and society* (2nd ed.). New York: Norton.

Exner, J. E., Jr. (2003). *The Rorschach: A comprehensive system* (4th ed.). New York: Wiley.

Exner, J. E., Jr., & Erdberg, P. (2002). Why use personality tests?: A brief history and some comments. In J. N. Butcher (Ed.), *Clinical personality assessment: Practical approaches* (2nd ed., pp. 7–12). London: Oxford University Press.

Eysenck, H. J. (1952). *The scientific study of personality.* London: Routledge & Kegan Paul.

Eysenck, H. J. (1973). *Eysenck on extraversion.* New York: Wiley.

Eysenck, H. J. (1990). Biological dimensions of personality. In L. Pervin (Ed.), *Handbook of personality: Theory and research* (pp. 244–276). New York: Guilford Press.

Fairbairn, W. R. D. (1954). *An object relations theory of the personality.* New York: Basic Books.

Farrell, A. G., & Sullivan, T. N. (2000). Structure of the Weinberger Adjustment Inventory Self-Restraint scale and its relation to problem behaviors in adolescence. *Psychological Assessment, 4,* 394–401.

Fine, R. (1990). *Love and work: The value system of psychoanalysis.* New York: Continuum.

Fonagy, P., & Target, M. (1996). Playing with reality I: Theory of mind and the normal development of psychic reality. *International Journal of Psychoanalysis, 77,* 217–233.

Fonagy, P., Moran, G. S., Steele, M., Steele, H., & Higgitt, A. C. (1991). The capacity for understanding mental states: The reflective self in parent and child and its significance for security of attachment. *Infant Mental Health Journal, 13,* 200–216.

Foucault, M. (1977). *Discipline and punish: The birth of the prison.* New York: Pantheon Books.

Frankl, V. (1963). *Man's search for meaning.* Boston: Beacon.

Frazier, C. (2003). *Cold mountain.* London: Sceptre Paperbacks. (Original work published 1997)

Freud, A. (1936). *The ego and the mechanisms of defense.* New York: International Universities Press.

Freud, S. (1953). Repression. In J. Strachey (Ed. & Trans.), *The standard edition of the complete psychological works of Sigmund Freud* (Vol. 14, pp. 141–158). (Original work published 1915)

Fromm, E. (1941). *Escape from freedom.* New York: Rinehart & Company.

Gadamer, H. G. (1975). *Truth and method.* New York: Seabury Press.

Galton, F. (1884). Measurement of character. *Fortnightly Review, 36,* 179–185.

Gangestad, S. W., & Simpson, J. A. (2000). The evolution of human mating: Trade-offs and strategic pluralism. *Behavioral and Brain Sciences, 23,* 573–587.

Garner, E. H., Steiner, H., Huckaby, W. J., & Kohler, M. (1998). A comparison between the Weinberger Adjustment Inventory and the Minnesota Multiphasic Personality Inventory with incarcerated adolescent males. *Child Psychiatry and Human Development, 28,* 273–285.

Geertz, C. (1984). "From the native's point of view": On the nature of anthropological understanding. In R. A. Shweder & R. A. Levine (Eds.), *Culture theory: Essays on mind, self, and emotion* (pp. 123–136). Cambridge, UK: Cambridge University Press.

Gergen, K. J. (1991). *The saturated self: Dilemmas of identity in contemporary life.* New York: Basic Books.

Glassman, N. S., & Andersen, S. M. (1999). Streams of thought about the self and significant others: Transference as the construction of interpersonal meaning. In J. A. Singer & P. Salovey (Eds.), *At play in the fields of consciousness: Essays in honor of Jerome L. Singer* (pp. 103–140). Mahwah, NJ: Erlbaum.

Goldberg, L. R. (1981). Language and individual differences: The search for universals in personality lexicons. In L. Wheeler (Ed.), *Review of personality and social psychology* (Vol. 2, pp. 141–165). Beverly Hills, CA: Sage.

Goldberg, L. R. (1982). From Ace to Zombie: Some explorations in the language of personality. In C. D. Spielberger & J. N. Butcher (Eds.), *Advances in personality assessment* (Vol. 1, pp. 203–234). Hillsdale, NJ: Erlbaum.

Goldberg, L. R. (1990). An alternative "description of personality": The big-five factor structure. *Journal of Personality and Social Psychology, 59,* 1216–1229.

Gosling, S. D., & John, O. P. (1999). Personality dimensions in nonhuman animals: A cross-species review. *Current Directions in Psychological Science, 8,* 69–75.

Greenberg, G. (1994). *Self on the shelf: Recovery books and the good life.* Albany: State University of New York Press.

Greenberg, G. (1995). If a self is a narrative: Social constructionism in the clinic. *Journal of Narrative and Life History, 5,* 269–283.

Greenberg, G. (March, 2004). After nature: The varieties of technological experience. *Harper's Magazine,* pp. 91–96.

Greenberg, L. S. (2002). *Emotion-focused therapy: Coaching clients to work through their feelings.* Washington, DC: American Psychological Association.

Greenberg, L. S., & Angus, L. E. (2004). The contributions of emotional processes to narrative change in psychotherapy: A dialectical constructivist approach.

In L. E. Angus & J. McLeod (Eds.), *The handbook of narrative and psychotherapy* (pp. 331–349). Thousand Oaks, CA: Sage.

Guisinger, S. (2003). Adapted to flee famine: Adding an evolutionary perspective on anorexia nervosa. *Psychological Review, 110,* 745–761.

Harlow, H. F. (1958). The nature of love. *American Psychologist, 13,* 673–685.

Harlow, H. F., & Harlow, M. K. (1962). The effect of rearing conditions on behavior. *Bulletin of the Menninger Clinic, 26,* 213–224.

Harlow, H. F., & Zimmerman, R. R. (1959). Affectional responses in the infant monkey. *Science, 130,* 421–432.

Hart, D., Hofmann, V., Edelstein, W., & Keller, M. (1997). The relation of childhood personality types to adolescent behavior and development: A longitudinal study of Icelandic children. *Developmental Psychology, 33,* 195–205.

Hegelson, V. S., & Fritz, H. L. (2000). The implications of unmitigated agency and unmitigated communion for domains of problem behavior. *Journal of Personality, 68,* 1031–1057.

Hendrix, H. (1988). *Getting the love you want: A couples guide.* New York: Henry Holt.

Hermans, H. J. M. (1996). Voicing the self: From information processing to dialogical interchange. *Psychological Bulletin, 119,* 31–50.

Higgins, E. T. (1987). Self-discrepancy: A theory relating self and affect. *Psychological Review, 94,* 319–340.

Higgins, E. T. (1997). Beyond pain and pleasure. *American Psychologist, 52,* 1280–1300.

Higgins, E. T. (1998). Promotion and prevention: Regulatory focus as a motivational principle. *Advances in Experimental Social Psychology, 30,* 1–46.

Horowitz, M. J. (1991). (Ed). *Person schemas and maladaptive interpersonal patterns.* Chicago: University of Chicago Press.

Inhelder, B., & Piaget, J. (1958). *The growth of logical thinking from childhood to adolescence.* New York: Basic Books.

Jackson, D. N. (1974). *The Personality Research Form.* Port Huron, MI: Research Psychologists Press.

Jacobson, E. (1964). *The self and the object world.* New York: International Universities Press.

John, O. P., & Srivastava, S. (1999). The Big Five trait taxonomy: History, measurement, and theoretical perspectives. In L. A. Pervin & O. P. John (Eds.), *Handbook of personality: Theory and research* (2nd ed., pp. 102–138). New York: Guilford Press.

Josephson, B., Singer, J. A., & Salovey, P. (1996). Mood regulation and memory: Repairing sad moods with happy memories. *Cognition and Emotion, 10,* 437–444.

Josselson, R. (1996). *Revising herself: The story of women's identity from college to midlife.* New York: Oxford University Press.

Josselson, R., Lieblich, A., & McAdams, D. P. (Eds.). (2003). *Up close and personal: The teaching and learning of narrative research.* Washington, DC: American Psychological Association Books.

Karon, B. P. (2000). The clinical interpretation of the Thematic Apperception Test,

Rorschach, and other clinical data: A reexamination of statistical versus clinical prediction. *Professional Psychology: Research and Practice, 31,* 230–233.

Kegan, R. (1982). *The evolving self: Problem and process in human development.* Cambridge, MA: Harvard University Press.

Kiesler, D. J. (1996). *Contemporary interpersonal theory and research: Personality, psychopathology, and psychotherapy.* New York: Wiley.

Kiesler, D. J. (2002). *Contemporary interpersonal theory and research: Personality, psychopathology, and psychotherapy* (2nd ed.). New York: Wiley.

Kiesler, D. J., & Schmidt, J. A. (1993). *The Impact Message Inventory: Form IIA Octant Scale version.* Palo Alto, CA: Mind Garden.

Kihlstrom, J. F. (1981). On personality and memory. In N. Cantor & J. F. Kihlstrom (Eds.), *Personality, cognition, and social interaction* (pp. 123–179). Hillsdale, NJ: Erlbaum.

Kihlstrom, J. F. (1987). The cognitive unconscious. *Science, 237,* 1445–1452.

King, L. A. (1995). Wishes, motives, goals, and personal memories: Relations of measures of human motivation. *Journal of Personality, 63,* 985–1007.

King, L. A., & Raspin, C. K. (2004). Lost and possible selves, subjective well-being, and ego development in divorced women. *Journal of Personality, 72,* 603–632.

King, L. A., Scollon, C. K., Ramsey, C., & May, T. (2000). Stories of life transition: Subjective well-being and ego development in parents of children with Down Syndrome. *Journal of Research in Personality, 34,* 509–536.

Klein, M. (1975). *Envy and gratitude and other works, 1946–1963.* New York: Delacorte Press.

Klinger, E. (1999). Thought flow: Properties and mechanisms underlying shifts in content. In J. A. Singer & P. Salovey (Eds.), *At play in the fields of consciousness: Essays in honor of Jerome L. Singer* (pp. 29–50). Mahwah, NJ: Erlbaum.

Knapp, P. H. (1991). Self–other schemas: Core organizers of human experience. In M. Horowitz (Ed.), *Person schemas and maladaptive interpersonal patterns* (pp. 81–102). Chicago: University of Chicago Press.

Koestner, R., Weinberger, J., & McClelland, D. C. (1991). Task-intrinsic and social-extrinsic sources of arousal for motives assessed in fantasy and self-report. *Journal of Personality, 59,* 57–82.

Kohut, H. (1971). *The analysis of the self.* New York: International Universities Press.

Kretschmer, E. (1921). *Korperbau und charakter* [Physique and character]. Berlin: Springer.

Lamiell, J. T. (2003). *Beyond individual and group differences.* Thousand Oaks, CA: Sage.

Lanning, K. (1994). Dimensionality of observer ratings on the California Adult Q-Set. *Journal of Personality and Social Psychology, 67,* 151–160.

Lau, B. (2002). The Prelude and self-defining memories. In L. H. Peer (Ed.), *Recent perspectives on European romanticism* (pp. 99–103). Lewiston, NY: Edwin Mellen.

Leary, T. F. (1957). *Interpersonal diagnosis of personality.* New York: Ronald.

LeDoux, J. (1996). *The emotional brain.* New York: Simon & Schuster.

Levenson, E. A. (1991). *The purloined self: Interpersonal perspectives in psycho-analysis.* New York: William Alanson White Institute.

Lieblich, A., McAdams, D. P., & Josselson, R. (Eds.). (2004). *Healing plots: The narrative basis of psychotherapy.* Washington, DC: American Psychological Association Books.

Lilienfeld, S. O., Wood, J. M., & Garb, H. N. (2000). The scientific status of projective techniques. *Psychological Science in the Public Interest, 1,* 27–66.

Linehan, M. M. (1988). Perspectives on the interpersonal relationship in behavior therapy. *Journal of Integrative and Eclectic Psychotherapy, 7,* 278–290.

Little, B. R. (1989). Personal projects analysis: Trivial pursuits, magnificent obsessions, and the search for coherence. In D. M. Buss & N. Cantor (Eds.), *Personality psychology: Recent trends and emerging directions* (pp. 15–31). New York: Springer-Verlag.

Little, B. R. (1999). Personality and motivation: Personal action and the conative evolution. In L. A. Pervin & O. P. John (Eds.), *Handbook of personality: Theory and research* (2nd ed., pp. 501–524). New York: Guilford Press.

Loehlin, J. C., McCrae, R. R., Costa, P. T., Jr., & John, O. P. (1998). Heritabilities of common and measure-specific components of the Big Five personality factors. *Journal of Research in Personality, 32,* 431–453.

Loevinger, J. (1976). *Ego development.* San Francisco: Jossey-Bass.

Loevinger, J. (1983). On ego development and the structure of personality. *Developmental Review, 3,* 339–350.

Luborsky, L. (1990). A guide to the CCRT method. In L. Luborsky & P. Crits-Christoph (Eds.), *Understanding transference: The Core Conflictual Relationship Theme method* (pp. 15–36). New York: Basic Books.

Luborsky, L. (1997). The Core Conflictual Relationship Theme (CCRT): A basic case formulation method. In T. D. Eells (Ed.), *Handbook of psychotherapy case formulation* (pp. 58–83). New York: Guilford Press.

Luborsky, L. (1998). The early life of the idea for the Core Conflictual Relationship Theme method. In L. Luborsky & P. Crits-Christoph (Eds.), *Understanding transference: The core conflictual relationship theme method* (2nd ed., pp. 3–14). Washington, DC: American Psychological Association.

Luborsky, L., & Crits-Christoph, P. (Eds.). (1998). *Understanding transference: The core conflictual relationship theme method* (2nd ed.). Washington, DC: American Psychological Association Press.

MacIntyre, A. (1981). *After virture: A study in moral theory.* Notre Dame, IN: University of Notre Dame Press.

Mahler, M. S. (1968). *On human symbiosis and the vicissitudes of individuation: Infantile psychosis.* New York: International Universities Press.

Mahoney, M. J. (2003). *Constructive psychotherapy: A practical guide.* New York: Guilford Press.

Main, M. (1983). Exploration, play, and cognitive functioning related to mother–infant attachment. *Infant Behavior and Development, 6,* 167–174.

Main, M., Kaplan, N., & Cassidy, J. (1985). Security in infancy, childhood, and adulthood: A move to the level of representation. *Monographs of the Society for Research in Child Development, 50* (1 & 2), 66–104.

Marcia, J. E. (1966). Development and validation of ego identity status. *Journal of Personality and Social Psychology, 3,* 551–558.

Marcia, J. E. (1980). Identity in adolescence. In J. Adelson (Ed.), *Handbook of adolescent psychology* (pp. 159–187). New York: Wiley.

Markus, H. (1977). Self-schemata and processing information about the self. *Journal of Personality and Social Psychology, 35,* 63–78.

Markus, H. (1983). Self-knowledge: An expanded view. *Journal of Personality, 51,* 543–565.

Markus, H., & Kitayama, S. (1991). Culture and the self: Implications for cognition, emotion, and motivation. *Psychological Review, 98,* 224–253.

Maslow, A. H. (1987). *Motivation and personality.* New York: Harper & Row. (Original work published 1954)

Matt, G. E., Vazquez, C., & Campbell, W. K. (1992). Mood-congruent recall of affectively toned stimuli: A meta-analytic review. *Clinical Psychology Review, 12,* 227–255.

McAdams, D. P. (1980). A thematic coding system for the intimacy motive. *Journal of Research in Personality, 14,* 413–432.

McAdams, D. P. (1982). Experiences of intimacy and power: Relationships between social motives and autobiographical memory. *Journal of Personality and Social Psychology, 42,* 292–302.

McAdams, D. P. (1984). Scoring manual for the intimacy motive. *Psychological Documents, 14* (No. 2613), 7.

McAdams, D. P. (1987). A life story model of identity. In R. Hogan & W. H. Jones (Eds.), *Perspectives in personality* (Vol 2., pp. 15–50). Greenwich, CT: JAI Press.

McAdams, D. P. (1988). *Power, intimacy, and the life story: Personological inquiries into identity.* New York: Guilford Press.

McAdams, D. P. (1990). Unity and purpose in human lives: The emergence of identity as a life story. In A. I. Rabin, R. A. Zucker, R. A. Emmons, & S. Frank (Eds.), *Studying persons and lives* (pp. 148–200). New York: Springer.

McAdams, D. P. (1993). *The stories we live by: Personal myths and the making of the self.* New York: Morrow.

McAdams, D. P. (1995). What do we know when we know a person? *Journal of Personality, 63,* 365–396.

McAdams, D. P. (1996). Personality, modernity, and the storied self: A contemporary framework for studying persons. *Psychological Inquiry, 7,* 295–321.

McAdams, D. P. (1997). A conceptual history of personality psychology. In R. Hogan, J. Johnson, & S. Briggs (Eds.), *Handbook of personality psychology* (pp. 3–39). San Diego: Academic Press.

McAdams, D. P. (1999). Personal narratives and the life story. In L. A. Pervin & O. P. John (Eds.), *Handbook of personality: Theory and research* (2nd ed., pp. 478–500). New York: Guilford Press.

McAdams, D. P. (2001). The psychology of life stories. *Review of General Psychology, 5,* 100–122.

McAdams, D. P. (2002). Coding autobiographical episodes for themes of agency and communion. Available on the Foley Center for the Study of Lives website: www. sesp.northwestern.edu/foley

McAdams, D. P. (2006). *The person: A new introduction to personality psychology* (4th ed.). Forth Worth, TX: Harcourt.

McAdams, D. P., & de St. Aubin, E. (1992). A theory of generativity and its assessment through self-report, behavioral acts, and narrative themes in autobiography. *Journal of Personality and Social Psychology, 62,* 1003–1015.

McAdams, D. P., Hoffman, B. J., Mansfield, E. D., & Day, R. (1996). Themes of agency and communion in significant autobiographical scenes. *Journal of Personality, 64,* 339–377.

McAdams, D. P., Josselson, R., & Lieblich, A. (Eds.). (2001). *Turns in the road: Narrative studies of lives in transition.* Washington, DC: American Psychological Association Books.

McAdams, D. P., Reynolds, J., Lewis, M., Patten, A. H., & Bowman, P. J. (2001). When bad things turn good and good things turn bad: Sequences of redemption and contamination in life narrative and their relation to psychosocial adaptation in midlife adults and in students. *Personality and Social Psychology Bulletin, 27,* 474–485.

McClelland, D. C. (1961). *The achieving society.* New York: D. Van Nostrand.

McClelland, D. C. (1985). *Human motivation.* Glenview, IL: Scott, Foresman.

McClelland, D. C., Koestner, R., & Weinberger, J. (1989). How do self-attributed and implicit motives differ? *Psychological Review, 96,* 690–702.

McCrae, R. R. (1996). Social consequences of experiential openness. *Psychological Bulletin, 120,* 323–337.

McCrae, R. R. (1993). Moderated analyses of longitudinal personality stability. *Journal of Personality and Social Psychology, 65,* 577–585.

McCrae, R. R., & Costa, P. T., Jr. (1985). Updating Norman's "adequate taxonomy": Intelligence and personality dimensions in natural language and in questionnaires. *Journal of Personality and Social Psychology, 49,* 710–721.

McCrae, R. R., & Costa, P. T., Jr. (1987). Validation of the five-factor model of personality across instruments and observers. *Journal of Personality and Social Psychology, 52,* 81–90.

McCrae, R. R., & Costa, P. T., Jr. (1989). Different points of view: Self-reports and ratings in the assessment of personality. In J. P. Forgas & M. J. Innes (Eds.), *Recent advances in social psychology; An international perspective* (pp. 429–439). Amsterdam: Elsevier.

McCrae, R. R., & Costa, P. T., Jr. (1990). *Personality in adulthood.* New York: Guilford Press.

McCrae, R. R., & Costa, P. T., Jr. (1991). Adding *Liebe und arbeit:* The full five-factor model and well-being. *Personality and Social Psychology Bulletin, 17,* 227–232.

McCrae, R. R., & Costa, P. T., Jr. (1997). Personality trait structure as a human universal. *American Psychologist, 52,* 509–516.

McCrae, R. R., & Costa, P. T., Jr. (1999). A five-factor theory of personality. In L. A. Pervin & O. P. John (Eds.), *Handbook of personality: Theory and research* (2nd ed., pp. 139–153). New York: Guilford Press.

McCrae, R. R., & Costa, P. T, Jr. (2003). *Personality in adulthood: A five-factor theory perspective* (2nd ed.). New York: Guilford Press.

McCrae, R. R., Costa, P. T., Jr., del Pilar, G. H., Rolland, J. P., & Parker, W. D.

(1998). Cross-cultural assessment of the five-factor model: The Revised NEO Personality Inventory. *Journal of Cross-Cultural Psychology, 29,* 171–188.

McCrae, R. R., Costa, P. T., Jr., Lima, M. P., Simoes, A., Ostendorf, F., Angleitner, A., Marusic, I., Bratko, D., Caprara, G. V., Barbaranelli, C., Chae, J. H., & Piedmont, R. L. (1999). Age differences in personality across the adult lifespan: Parallels in five cultures. *Developmental Psychology, 35,* 466–477.

McCrae, R. R., Costa, P. T., Jr., Ostendorf, F., Angleitner, A., Hrebickova, M., Avia, M. D., Sanz, J., Sanchez-Bernardos, M. L., Kusdil, M. E., Woodfield, R., Saunders, P. R., & Smith, P. B. (2000). Nature over nurture: Temperament, personality, and lifespan development. *Journal of Personality and Social Psychology, 78,* 173–186.

McCrae, R. R., & John, O. P. (1992). An introduction to the five-factor model and its applications. *Journal of Personality, 60,* 175–215.

McCrae, R. R., Stone, S. V., Fagan, P. J., & Costa, P. T., Jr. (1998). Identifying causes of disagreement between self-reports and spouse ratings of personality. *Journal of Personality, 66,* 285–313.

Millon, T., Davis, R., & Millon, C. (1997). *MCMI-III manual.* Minneapolis, MN: National Computer Systems.

Milton, J. (2001). *The road to malpsychia: Humanistic psychology and its discontents.* San Francisco: Encounter Books.

Mischel, W. (1968). *Personality and assessment.* New York: Wiley.

Mischel, W., & Schoda, Y. (1999). Integrating dispositions and processing dynamics within a unified theory of personality: The cognitive–affective personality system. In L. A. Pervin & O. P. John (Eds.), *Handbook of personality: Theory and research* (2nd ed., pp. 197–218). New York: Guilford Press.

Mischel, W., Shoda, Y., & Mendoza-Denton, R. (2002). Situation-behavior profiles as a locus of consistency in personality. *Current Directions in Psychological Science, 11,* 50–54.

Misiak, H., & Sexton, V. S. (1973). *Phenomenological, existential, and humanistic psychologies: A historical survey.* New York: Grune & Stratton.

Mitchell, S. A. (1988). *Relational concepts in psychoanalysis.* Cambridge, MA: Harvard University Press.

Mitchell, S. A. (2000). *Relationality: From attachment to intersubjectivity.* Hillsdale, NJ: Analytic Press.

Moffitt, K. H., & Singer, J. A. (1994). Continuity in the life story: Self-defining memories, affect, and approach/avoidance personal strivings. *Journal of Personality, 62,* 21–43.

Moffitt, K. H., Singer, J. A., Nelligan, D. W., Carlson, M. A., & Vyse, S. A. (1994). Depression and memory narrative type. *Journal of Abnormal Psychology, 103,* 581–583.

Moore, R. G., Watts, F. N., & Williams, J. M. G. (1988). The specificity of personal memories in depression. *British Journal of Clinical Psychology, 27,* 275–276.

Moss, D. (2001). The roots and genealogy of humanistic psychology. In K. J. Schneider, J. F. T. Bugental, & J. F. Pierson (Eds.), *The handbook of humanistic psychology: Leading edges in theory, research, and practice* (pp. 5–20). Thousand Oaks, CA: Sage.

Murray, H. A. (1938). *Explorations in personality.* New York: Oxford University Press.

Murray, H. A. (1943). *The Thematic Apperception Test: Manual.* Cambridge, MA: Harvard University Press.

Nelson, K., & Fivush, R. (2004). The emergence of autobiographical memory: A social cultural developmental theory. *Psychological Review, 111,* 486–511.

Nicholson, I. A. (2003). *Inventing personality: Gordon Allport and the science of selfhood.* Washington, DC: American Psychological Association Books.

Norman, W. T. (1963). Toward an adequate taxonomy of personality attributes: Replicated factor structure in peer nomination personality ratings. *Journal of Abnormal and Social Psychology, 66,* 574–583.

Ogden, T. H. (1991). *Projective identification and psychotherapeutic technique.* Northvale, NJ: Aronson.

Ogden, T. H. (1994). The analytic third: Working with intersubjective clinical facts. *International Journal of Psycho-Analysis, 75,* 3–19.

Ogden, T. H. (2004). The analytic third: Implications for psychoanalytic theory and technique. *Psychoanalytic Quarterly, 73,* 167–195.

Ogilvie, D. M., & Ashmore, R. D. (1991). Self-with-other representation as a unit of analysis in self-concept research. In R. A. Curtis (Ed.), *The relational self: Theoretical convergences in psychoanalysis and social psychology* (pp. 282–314). New York: Guilford Press.

Ogilvie, D. M., Fleming, C. J., & Pennell, G. E. (1998). Self-with-other representations. In D. F. Barone, M. Hersen, & V. B. Van Hasselt (Eds.), *Advanced personality* (pp. 353–376). New York: Plenum Press.

Pasupathi, M. (2001). The social construction of the personal past and its implications for adult development. *Psychological Bulletin, 127,* 651–672.

Pennebaker, J. W. (Ed.). (1995). *Emotion, disclosure, and health.* Washington DC: American Psychological Association.

Pennebaker, J. W. (1997). Writing about emotional experiences as a therapeutic process. *Psychological Science, 8,* 162–166.

Pennebaker, J. W., & Francis, M. E. (1996). Cognitive, emotional, and language processes in disclosure. *Cognition and Emotion, 10,* 601–626.

Pennebaker, J. W., & Keough, K. A. (1999). Revealing, organizing, and reorganizing the self in response to stress and emotion. *Self, Social Identity, and Physical Health, 2,* 101–121.

Pennebaker, J. W., & Seagal, J. D. (1999). Forming a story: The health benefits of a narrative. *Journal of Clinical Psychology, 55,* 1243–1254.

Pervin, L. A., & John, O. P. (Eds.). (1999). *Handbook of personality: Theory and research* (2nd ed.). New York: Guilford Press.

Phillips, K. A. (2001). Body dysmorphic disorder. In K. A. Phillips (Ed.), *Review of psychiatry: Vol. 20. Somatoform and factitious disorders* (pp. 67–94). Washington, DC: American Psychiatric Association.

Piedmont, R. L. (1998). *The Revised NEO Personality Inventory: Clinical and research applications.* New York: Plenum Press.

Pillemer, D. B. (1998). *Momentous events, vivid memories.* Cambridge, MA: Harvard University Press.

Pillemer, D. B. (2001). Momentous events and the life story. *Review of General Psychology, 5,* 123–134.

Pillemer, D. B., Rhinehart, E. D., & White, S. H. (1986). Memories of life transitions: The first year in college. *Human Learning, 5,* 109–123.

Pinker, S. (1999). *How the mind works.* New York: Norton.

Plato. (1953). *The Dialogues of Plato.*(B. Jowett Trans.), Oxford, UK: Clarendon Press.

Popper, K. (1959). *The logic of scientific discovery.* New York: Basic Books.

Racker, H. (1968). *Transference and countertransference.* New York: International Universities Press.

Reynolds, S. K., & Clark, L. A. (2001). Predicting dimensions of personality disorder from domains and facets of the five-factor model. *Journal of Personality, 69,* 199–222.

Ricoeur, P. (1984). *Time and narrative 1* (Kathleen McGlaughlin & David Pellauer, Trans.) Chicago: University of Chicago Press.

Riemann, R., Angleitner, A., & Strelau, J. (1997). Genetic and environmental influences on personality: A study of twins reared together using the self- and peer-report NEO-FFI scales. *Journal of Personality, 65,* 449–475.

Robins, R. W., Fraley, R. C., Roberts, B. W., & Trzesniewski, K. H. (2001). A longitudinal study of personality change in young adulthood. *Journal of Personality, 69,* 617–640.

Robinson, D. (1976). *An intellectual history of psychology.* New York: Macmillan.

Robinson, F. G. (1992). *Love's story told: A life of Henry Murray.* Cambridge, MA: Harvard University Press.

Robinson, J. A. (1986). Autobiographical memory: A historical prologue. In D. C. Rubin (Ed.), *Autobiographical memory* (pp. 19–23). Cambridge, UK: Cambridge University Press.

Rodin, J., Silberstein, L., & Striegel-Moore, R. (1985). Women and weight: A normative discontent. In T. R. Sonderegger (Ed.), *Psychology and gender: Nebraska Symposium on Motivation: 1984.* Lincoln: University of Nebraska Press.

Rodman, F. R. (2003). *Winnicott: Life and work.* Cambridge, MA: Perseus.

Rogers, C. R. (1951). *Client-centered therapy.* Boston: Houghton Mifflin.

Rotter, J. B. (1966). Generalized expectancies for internal vs. external control of reinforcment. *Psychological Monographs, 80,* (1, Whole No. 609).

Rousseau, J.-J. (1953). *The confessions* (J. M. Cohen, Trans.). London: Penguin Books. (Original work published 1781)

Ruehlman, L. S., & Wolchik, S. A. (1988). Personal goals and interpersonal support and hindrance as factors in psychological distress and well-being. *Journal of Personality and Social Psychology, 55,* 293–301.

Runyan, W. M. (1982). *Life histories and psychobiography: Explorations in theory and method.* New York: Oxford University Press.

Runyan, W. M. (1997). Studying lives: Psychobiography and the conceptual structure of personality psychology. In R. Hogan, J. Johnson, & S. Briggs (Eds.), *Handbook of personality psychology* (pp. 41–69). San Diego: Academic Press.

Rusting, C. L. (1998). Personality, mood, and cognitive processing of emotional information: Three conceptual frameworks. *Psychological Bulletin, 124,* 165–196.

Sampson, E. E. (1988). The debate on individualism: Indigenous psychologies of the individual and their role in personal and societal functioning. *American Psychologist, 43,* 15–23.

Sandstrom, M. J., & Cramer, P. (2003a). Defense mechanisms and psychological adjustment in childhood. *Journal of Nervous and Mental Disease, 191,* 487–495.

Sandstrom, M. J., & Cramer, P. (2003b). Girls' use of defense mechanisms following peer rejection. *Journal of Personality, 71,* 605–627.

Sarbin, T. R. (1986). The narrative as a root metaphor for psychology. In T. R. Sarbin (Ed.), *Narrative psychology: The storied nature of human conduct* (pp. 3–21). New York: Praeger.

Saucier, G. (1997). Effects of variable selection on the factor structure of person descriptors. *Journal of Personality and Social Psychology, 73,* 1296–1312.

Saucier, G., & Goldberg, L. R. (1996). The language of personality: Lexical perspectives on the five-factor model. In J. S. Wiggins (Ed.), *The five-factor model of personality: Theoretical perspectives* (pp. 21–50). New York: Guilford Press.

Schafer, R. (1983). *The analytic attitude.* New York: Basic Books.

Schank, R. C., & Abelson, R. P. (1977). *Scripts, plans, goals, and understanding.* Hillsdale, NJ: Erlbaum.

Schenkel, S., & Marcia, J. E. (1972). Attitudes toward pre-marital intercourse in determining ego identity status in college women. *Journal of Personality, 3,* 472–482.

Schneider, K. J., Bugental, J. K., Pierson, J. F. (2001). *The handbook of humanistic psychology: Leading edges in theory, research, and practice.* Thousand Oaks, CA: Sage.

Schultheiss, O. C., & Brunstein, J. C. (1999). Goal imagery: Bridging the gap between implicit and explicit goals. *Journal of Personality, 67,* 1–37.

Schultz, W. T. (2003). The prototypical scene: A method for generating psychobiographical hypotheses. In R. Josselson, A. Lieblich, & D. P. McAdams (Eds.), *Up close and personal: The teaching and learning of narrative research* (pp. 151–175). Washington, DC: American Psychological Association.

Segal, Z. V., Williams, J. M. G., & Teasdale, J. D. (2001). *Mindfulness-based cognitive therapy for depression: A new approach to preventing relapse.* New York: Guilford Press.

Seligman, M. (2002). *Authentic happiness: Using the new positive psychology to realize your potential for lasting fulfillment.* New York: Free Press.

Sheldon, W. H. (1940). *The varieties of human physique: An introduction to constitutional psychology.* New York: Harper.

Shweder, R. A., & Bourne, E. J. (1985). Does the concept of the person vary cross-culturally? In R. A. Schweder & R. A. LeVine (Eds.), *Culture theory: Essays on mind, self, and emotion* (pp. 158–199). Cambridge, UK: Cambridge University Press.

Singer, J. A. (1990). Affective responses to autobiographical memories and their relationship to long-term goals. *Journal of Personality, 58,* 535–563.

Singer, J. A. (1995). Seeing one's self: Locating narrative memory in a framework of personality. *Journal of Personality, 51,* 206–231.

Singer, J. A. (1997). *Message in a bottle: Stories of men and addiction.* New York: Free Press.

Singer, J. A. (2001). Living in the amber cloud: A life story analysis of a heroin addict. In D. P. McAdams, R. Josselson, & A. Lieblich (Eds.), *Turns in the road: Narrative studies of lives in transition* (pp. 253–277). Washington, DC: American Psychological Association.

Singer, J. A. (2004a). A love story: Using self-defining memories in couples therapy. In D. P. McAdams, R. Josselson, & A. Lieblich (Eds.), *Healing plots: Narrative and psychotherapy.* Washington, DC: American Psychological Association.

Singer, J. A. (2004b). Narrative identity and meaning-making across the adult lifespan: An introduction to a special issue of the *Journal of Personality. Journal of Personality, 72,* 437–459.

Singer, J. A., & Blagov, P. S. (2002). *Classification system and scoring manual for self-defining autobiographical memories.* New London, CT: Department of Psychology, Connecticut College.

Singer, J. A., & Blagov, P. (2004a). The integrative function of narrative processing: Autobiographical memory, self-defining memories and the life story of identity. In D. Beike, J. Lampinen, & D. Behrend (Eds.), *Self and memory: Evolving concepts* (pp. 117–138). New York: Psychology Press.

Singer, J. A., & Blagov, P. S. (2004b). Self-defining memories, narrative identity, and psychotherapy: A conceptual model, empirical investigation, and case report. In L. E. Angus & J. McLeod (Eds.), *Handbook of narrative and psychotherapy: Practice, theory and research* (pp. 229–246). Thousand Oaks, CA: Sage.

Singer, J. A., King, L. A., Green, M. C., & Barr, S. C. (2002). Personal identity and civic responsibility: "Rising to the occasion" narratives and generativity in community action interns. *Journal of Social Issues, 58,* 535–556.

Singer, J. A., & Moffitt, K. H. (1991–1992). An experimental investigation of specificity and generality in memory narratives. *Imagination, Cognition and Personality, 11,* 233–257.

Singer, J. A., & Salovey, P. (1988). Mood and memory: Evaluating the network theory of affect. *Clinical Psychology Review, 8,* 211–251.

Singer, J. A., & Salovey, P. (1993). *The remembered self: Emotion and memory in personality.* New York: Free Press.

Singer, J. A., & Salovey, P. (1996). Motivated memory: Self-defining memories, goals, and affect regulation. In L. L. Martin & A. Tesser (Eds.), *Striving and feeling: Interactions among goals, affect, and self-regulation* (pp. 229–250). Hillsdale, NJ: Erlbaum.

Singer, J. A., & Singer, J. L. (1992). Transference in psychotherapy and daily life: Implications of current memory and social cognition research. In J. W. Barron & M. N. Eagle (Eds.), *Interface of psychoanalysis and psychology* (pp. 516–538). Washington, DC: American Psychological Association.

Singer, J. A., & Singer, J. L. (1994). Social-cognitive and narrative perspectives on transference. In J. M. Masling & R. F. Bornstein (Eds.), *Empirical perspectives on object relations theory: Empirical studies of psychoanalytic theories* (Vol. 5, pp. 157–193). Washington, DC: American Psychological Association.

Singer, J. L. (1984). The private personality. *Personality and Social Psychology Bulletin, 10,* 7–30.

Singer, J. L. (1988). Psychoanalytic theory in the context of contemporary psychology: The Helen Block Lewis memorial address. *Psychoanalytic Psychology, 5,* 95–125.

Singer, J. L., & Kolligian, J. (1987). Personality: Developments in the study of private experience. *Annual Review of Psychology, 38,* 533–574.

Smelser, N. J., & Erikson, E. H. (Eds.). (1980). *Themes of love and work in adulthood.* Cambridge, MA: Harvard University Press.

Smith, C. P. (Ed.). (1992). *Motivation and personality: Handbook of thematic content analysis.* New York: Cambridge University Press.

Smith, C. P. (2000). Content analysis and narrative analysis. In H. T. Reis & C. M. Judd (Eds.), *Handbook of research methods in social and personality psychology* (pp. 313–332). New York: Cambridge University Press.

Spence, D. P. (1982). *Narrative truth and historical truth.* New York: Norton.

Stahl, S. M., & Munter, N. (1999). *Essential psychopharmacology of depression and bipolar disorder.* Cambridge, UK: Cambridge University Press.

Staudinger, U. M. (2001). Life reflection: A social-cognitive analysis of life review. *Review of General Psychology, 5,* 148–160.

Staudinger, U. M., Lopez, D., & Baltes, P. B. (1997). The psychometric location of wisdom-related performance: Intelligence, personality, and more? *Personality and Social Psychology Bulletin, 23,* 1200–1214.

Steiner, H., & Feldman, S. S. (1995). Two approaches to the measurement of adaptive style: Comparison of normal, psychosomatically ill, and delinquent adolescents. *Journal of the American Academy of Child and Adolescent Psychiatry, 34,* 180–190.

Stern, D. N. (1985). *The interpersonal world of the infant: A view from psychoanalysis and developmental psychology.* New York: Basic Books.

Stolorow, R. D., & Atwood, G. E. (1992). *Contexts of being: The intersubjective foundations of psychological life.* Hillsdale, NJ: Analytic Press.

Stolorow, R. D., Atwood, G. E., & Ross, J. M. (1978). The representational world in psychoanalytic therapy. *International Review of Psychoanalysis, 5,* 247–256.

Sullivan, H. S. (1953). *The interpersonal theory of psychiatry.* New York: Norton.

Sullivan, H. S. (1954). *The psychiatric interview.* New York: Norton.

Sutin, A. R., & Robins, R. W. (2005). Continuity and correlates of emotions and motives in self-defining memories. *Journal of Personality, 73,* 793–824.

Taylor, C. (1989). *Sources of the self: The making of the modern identity.* Cambridge, MA: Harvard University Press.

Thorne, A. (1995). Developmental truths in memories of childhood and adolescence. *Journal of Personality, 63,* 138–163.

Thorne, A., Cutting, L., & Skaw, D. (1998). Young adults' relationship memories and the life story: Examples or essential landmarks. *Narrative Inquiry, 8*(2), 237–268.

Thorne, A., & Latzke, M. (1996). Contextualizing the storied self. *Psychological Inquiry, 7,* 372–376.

Thorne, A., & McLean, K. (2001). *Manual for coding events in self-defining memories.* Unpublished manuscript, Department of Psychology, University of California–Santa Cruz.

Thorne, A., McLean, K. C., & Lawrence A.M. (2004). When remembering is not enough: Reflecting on self-defining memories in late adolescence. *Journal of Personality, 72,* 513–541.

Thorne, A., & Michaelieu, Q. (1996). Situating adolescent gender and self-esteem with personal memories. *Child Development, 67,* 1374–1390.

Thornhill, R., & Palmer, C. T. (2000). *A natural history of rape.* Cambridge, MA: MIT Press.

Tomkins, S. S. (1962). *Affect, imagery, consciousness* (Vol. 1). New York: Springer.

Tomkins, S. S. (1963). *Affect, imagery, consciousness* (Vol. 2). New York: Springer.

Tomkins, S. S. (1979). Script theory: Differential magnification of affects. In H. E. Howe, Jr. & R. A. Dienstbier (Eds.), *Nebraska Symposium on Motivation 1978* (Vol. 26, pp. 201–236). Lincoln: University of Nebraska Press.

Tomkins, S. S. (1987). Script theory. In J. Aronoff, A. I. Rabin, & R. A. Zucker (Eds.), *The emergence of personality* (pp. 147–216). New York: Springer.

Trull, T. T. (1992). DSM-III-R personality disorders: Disorders and the five-factor model of personality: An empirical comparison. *Journal of Abnormal Psychology, 101,* 553–560.

Tupes, E. C., & Christal, R. C. (1961). *Recurrent personality factors based on trait ratings* (Technical Report No. ASD-TR-61-97). Lackland Air Force Base, TX: U.S. Air Force.

Turvey, C., & Salovey, P. (1993–1994). Measures of repression: Converging on the same construct? *Imagination, Cognition, and Personality, 13,* 279–289.

Vaillant, G. E. (1977). *Adaptation to life.* Boston: Little, Brown.

Vaillant, G. E. (1992). *Ego mechanisms of defense: A guide for clinicians and researchers.* Washington, DC: American Psychiatric Association Press.

Vaillant, G. E., & Drake, R. E. (1985). Maturity of defenses in relation to DSM-III Axis II personality disorder. *Archives of General Psychiatry, 42,* 597–601.

Vaillant, G. E., & McCullough, L. (1998). The role of ego mechanisms of defense in the diagnosis of personality disorders. In J. W. Barron (Ed.), *Making diagnosis meaningful: Enhancing evaluation and treatment of psychological disorders* (pp. 139–158). Washington, DC: American Psychological Association.

Vallacher, R. R., & Wegner, D. M. (1987). What do people think they're doing?: Action identification and human behavior. *Psychological Review, 94,* 3–15.

Voronov, M., & Singer, J. A. (2002). Filial piety reconsidered. *Journal of Social Psychology, 142,* 461–480.

Waterman, A. S. (1982). Identity development from adolescence to adulthood: An extension of theory and a review of research. *Developmental Psychology, 18,* 341–358.

Watson, D., & Clark, L. A. (1997). Extraversion and its positive emotional core. In

R. Hogan, J. Johnson, & S. Briggs (Eds.), *Handbook of personality psychology* (pp. 767–793). San Diego: Academic Press.

Watson, D., & Tellegen, A. (1985). Toward a consensual structure of mood. *Psychological Bulletin, 98,* 219–235.

Weinberger, D. A. (1995). The construct validity of the repressive coping style. In J. L. Singer (Ed.), *Repression and dissociation: Implications for personality theory, psychopathology, and health* (pp. 337–386). Chicago: University of Chicago Press.

Weinberger, D. A. (1997). Distress and self-restraint as measures of adjustment across the lifespan: Confirmatory factor analyses in clinical and nonclinical samples. *Psychological Assessment, 9,* 132–135.

Weinberger, D. A. (1998). Defenses, personality structure, and development: Integrating psychodynamic theory into a typological approach to personality. *Journal of Personality, 66,* 1061–1080.

Weinberger, D. A., & Davidson, M. N. (1994). Styles of inhibiting emotional expression: Distinguishing repressive coping from impression management. *Journal of Personality, 62,* 587–613.

Weinberger, D. A., & Schwartz, G. E. (1990). Distress and restraint as superordinate dimensions of self-reported adjustment: A typological perspective. *Journal of Personality, 58,* 381–417.

Wertz, F. J. (2001). Humanistic psychology and the qualitative research tradition. In K. J. Schneider, J. F. T. Bugental, & J. F. Pierson (Eds.), *The handbook of humanistic psychology: Leading edges in theory, research, and practice* (pp. 231–245). Thousand Oaks, CA: Sage.

Westen, D. (1991). Clinical assessment of object relations using the T.A.T. *Journal of Personality Assessment, 56,* 56–74.

Westen, D. (1995). A clinical–empirical model of personality: Life after the Mischelian Ice Age and the NEO-lithic era. *Journal of Personality, 63,* 496–523.

Westen, D. (1998). The scientific legacy of Sigmund Freud: Toward a psychodynamically informed psychological science. *Psychological Bulletin, 124,* 333–371.

Westen, D., & Morrison, K. (2001). A multidimensional meta-analysis of treatments for depression, panic, and generalized anxiety disorders: An empirical examination of empirically-supported therapies. *Journal of Consulting and Clinical Psychology, 69,* 875–899.

Westen, D., Muderrisoglu, S., Fowler, C., Shedler, J., & Koren, D. (1997). Affect regulation and affective experience: Individual differences, group differences, and measurement using a Q-sort procedure. *Journal of Consulting and Clinical Psychology, 65,* 429–439.

Westen, D., Novotny, C. M., & Thompson-Brenner, H. (2004). The empirical status of empirically-supported psychotherapies: Assumptions, findings and reporting in controlled clinical trials. *Psychological Bulletin, 130,* 631–663.

White, M. (2000). Re-engaging with history: The absent but implicit. In *Reflections on narrative practice: Essays and interviews*. Adelaide, Australia: Dulwich Centre Publications.

White, M. (2004). Folk psychology and narrative practice. In L. E. Angus & J.

McLeod (Eds.), *The handbook of narrative and psychotherapy* (pp. 15–51). Thousand Oaks, CA: Sage.

White, M., & Epston, D. (1990). *Narrative means to therapeutic ends.* New York: Norton.

Whitman, W. (1958). Song of myself. In *Leaves of Grass.* New York: Signet Classics. (Original work published 1891–1892)

Wiggins, J. S. (1979). A psychological taxonomy of trait descriptive terms: The interpersonal domain. *Journal of Personality and Social Psychology, 37,* 395–412.

Wiggins, J. S. (1982). Circumplex models of interpersonal behavior in clinical psychology. In P. C. Kendall & J. N. Butcher (Eds.), *Handbook of research in clinical psychology* (pp. 183–221). New York: Wiley.

Wiggins, J. S. (2003). *Paradigms of personality.* New York: Guilford Press.

Williams, J. M. G. (1996). Depression and the specificity of autobiographical memory. In D. C. Rubin (Ed.), *Remembering our past: Studies in autobiographical memory* (pp. 244–267). Cambridge, MA: Cambridge University Press.

Williams, J. M. G. (2004). Experimental cognitive psychology and clinical practice: Autobiographical memory as a paradigm case. In. J. Yiend (Ed.), *Cognition, emotion, and psychopathology* (pp. 251–269). Cambridge, UK: Cambridge University Press.

Williams, J. M. G., & Broadbent, K. (1986). Autobiographical memory in suicide attempters. *Journal of Abnormal Psychology, 95,* 144–149.

Williams, J. M. G., & Dritschel, B. H. (1988). Emotional disturbance and the specificity of autobiographical memory. *Cognition and Emotion, 2*(3), 221–234.

Williams, J. M. G., & Scott, J. (1988). Autobiographical memory in depression. *Psychological Medicine, 18,* 689–695.

Winnicott, D. W. (1965). The theory of the parent–infant relationship. In *The maturational processes and the facilitating environment: Studies in the theory of emotional development* (pp. 37–55). London: Hogarth Press. (Original work published 1960)

Winnicott, D. W. (1965). A personal view of the Kleinian contribution. In *The maturational processes and the facilitating environment: Studies in the theory of emotional development* (pp. 171–178). London: Hogarth Press. (Original work published 1962)

Winter, D. G. (1973). *The power motive.* New York: Free Press.

Witkin, H. A. (1950). Individual differences in ease of perception of embedded figures. *Journal of Personality, 19,* 1–15.

Woike, B. A. (1995). Most-memorable experiences: Evidence for a link between implicit and explicit motives and social cognitive processes in everyday life. *Journal of Personality and Social Psychology, 68,* 1081–1091.

Woike, B. A., Gersekovich, I., Piorkowski, R., & Polo, M. (1999). The role of motives in the content and structure of autobiographical memory. *Journal of Personality and Social Psychology, 76,* 600–612.

Woike, B. A., & Polo, M. (2001). Motive-related memories: Content, structure and affect. *Journal of Personality, 69,* 391–415.

Woody, S. R., & Sanderson, W. C. (Eds.). (1998). *Manuals for empirically sup-*

ported treatments—1998 update. Unpublished resource list available through Division 12 of the American Psychological Association, Washington, DC.

Wordsworth, W. (1984). The tables turned. In S. Gill (Ed.), *William Wordsworth: A critical edition of the major works.* Oxford, UK: Oxford University Press. (Original work published 1798)

Wright, J. C., & Zakriski, A. L. (2003). When syndromal similarity obscures functional dissimilarity: Distinctive evoked environments of externalizing and mixed syndrome boys. *Journal of Consulting and Clinical Psychology, 71,* 516–527.

Yalom, I. D. (1980). *Existential psychotherapy.* New York: Basic Books.

Zuroff, D. (1986). Was Gordon Allport a trait theorist? *Journal of Personality and Social Psychology, 51,* 993–1000.

Index